Wall Pilates Workouts For Women

Illustrated Step-by-Step Workouts and Video Tutorials for Beginners
and Seniors to Gain Flexibility, Strength and Balance

By Tonia O'Neal

What Does This Book Include?

Theoretical Introduction with Practical Advice: Discover the principles of Wall Pilates and how to apply them.

50+ Exercises with Textual Explanation and Detailed Illustrations: Each exercise is clearly described and illustrated to guide your practice.

QR Code Access to 80+ Workout Videos: Instantly access extensive video demonstrations to enhance your understanding and execution of each movement.

As promised, that's not all. Your purchase also grants you access to these valuable bonuses:

First Bonus: Extensive Video Library

Over 80 video recordings of the exercises in the book, enhancing your learning experience.

Second Bonus: 28-Day Wall Pilates Challenge

A comprehensive day-by-day guide to deepen your practice and improve your Pilates skills.

Third Bonus: Free eBook "Optimal Nutrition for Wall Pilates"

Learn how to support your training with nutritional advice tailored specifically for Wall Pilates.

With the purchase of this book, you will have everything you need to effectively integrate Wall Pilates into your routine, supported by expert guidance and comprehensive resources.

Scan QR to Download your Free eBook

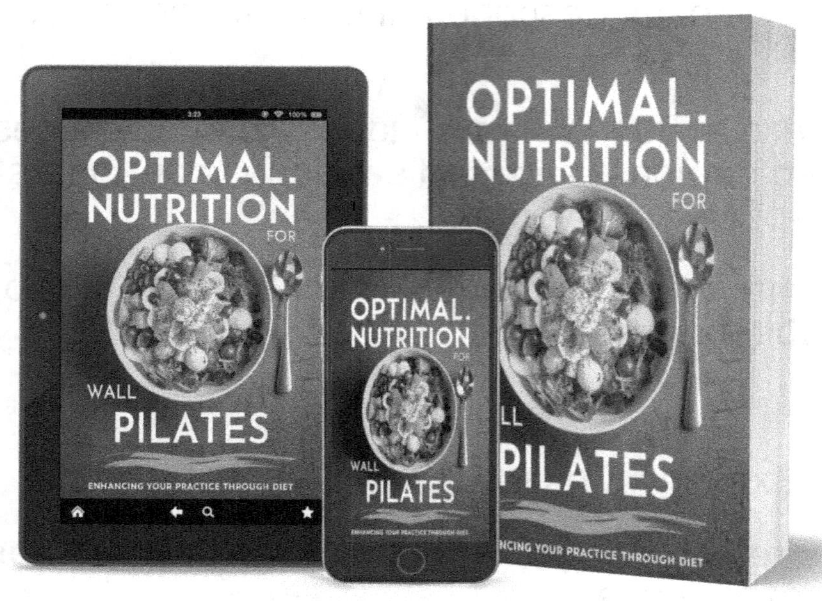

OR go to

https://peakform.gumroad.com/l/wallpilatesnutrition

Table of Contents

Introduction

As Janet leaned against the wall, catching her breath, she had a revelation. She had been attending the usual Pilates sessions for years, doing the same exercises on a mat with an increasing feeling of monotony. But this? This was different. The wall she was leaning on had transformed from a mere structural element of the room into her most supportive partner in fitness. In just a short time, she felt the areas of her body she'd neglected for years waking up, reminding her of the strength she once had in her youth. This was Wall Pilates, and it was about to change her life.

A recent study revealed that 75% of women over 40 and 85% of seniors believe that most mainstream fitness regimens don't cater to their specific needs. As the numbers suggest, this isn't a problem faced by a mere few. The world of fitness has often placed the spotlight on younger populations, leaving women over 40 and seniors searching in the dark for solutions tailored to their unique needs.

Are you one of the countless women or seniors who have felt the sting of exclusion in conventional exercise plans? Have you been searching for a fitness routine that understands the challenges of age, mobility, and changing bodily needs? You're not alone. From the searing pain of an old injury that flares up every time you try a new activity to the frustration of not finding exercise routines tailored to the nuances of your body, these problems aren't isolated — they're a shared struggle.

But what if there was a way to reclaim the strength, vitality, and confidence you once felt, or perhaps discover it for the first time? This isn't just about fitness. It's about rediscovering a part of yourself that you thought was lost to the sands of time. It's about recognizing that age doesn't define your potential; it simply redirects it. And with Wall Pilates, you're about to embark on a transformative journey that aligns with who you are, right here and now.

As you dive deeper into this book, your journey will take a clear and guided path. This isn't just a collection of exercises, but a 21-day program that's structured to evolve with you. Starting with the basics, you will first grasp the core principles of Wall Pilates. This foundational knowledge will ensure that each subsequent exercise and technique is effective, safe, and beneficial.

From the strength-focused practices that help in toning muscles to flexibility routines that enhance joint health, you're in for a holistic approach. But we don't stop there. Recognizing that our body's health is as much about what we eat as what we do, this guide intertwines its fitness teachings with a tailored nutrition plan. By understanding the synergistic relationship between diet and exercise, you will not only feel the changes but see them too.

So, why invest your time and energy in this book?

- Personalized Approach: This book has been meticulously designed with women and seniors in mind. This means exercises that respect and acknowledge your body's strengths and vulnerabilities, ensuring you get the most out of each session without risk of injury.
- Holistic Wellness: More than just physical exercises, this guide embraces a holistic approach. With the incorporation of a nutritional plan, you're not just working on external strength and flexibility, but also nurturing your body from the inside out.
- Empowerment and Independence: As you progress through the chapters, you will regain a sense of control over your health and well-being. Each exercise, each meal recommendation, is a step towards a more independent, agile, and confident you.
- Clear, Illustrative Guidance: With detailed photographs accompanying each exercise, there's no second-guessing. You will know precisely how to execute each move, ensuring effectiveness and safety.
- Adaptable Techniques: While this is a 21-day guide, the techniques and lessons you will learn are for life. Whether you wish to repeat the program, adapt it, or even integrate it with other fitness routines you love, the versatility of Wall Pilates is boundless.

You might be wondering, "Why should I trust this author to guide me through this transformative journey?" It's a valid question, and one I don't take lightly. Let me share a bit about myself so you can understand why I'm not just an author but a companion in this venture.

Several years ago, I found myself standing in your shoes, staring at a myriad of fitness programs and feeling none were made for me. Every crunch, jump, and sprint seemed like it was designed for someone else—someone younger, more agile, or without the nagging back pain that had been my uninvited companion for years. I was searching for a way to feel alive again, to feel capable again. That's when Wall Pilates entered my life, and nothing was ever the same.

I began incorporating Wall Pilates into my daily routine and felt like I was awakening muscles that had long been dormant. Over time, my posture improved, my aches lessened, and a newfound sense of vitality washed over me. That's when I realized this couldn't remain a personal secret; it had to be shared.

But I didn't just want to write a 'how-to' book; there are plenty of those. I wanted to write a 'how-to-for-YOU' book, one that recognized the unique challenges and opportunities that come with being a woman over 40 or a senior. That's why I delved deep into studying how Wall Pilates could specifically benefit these groups. I consulted experts, researched extensively, and tested the routines you're about to learn on myself and others in our demographic. The exercises and nutritional plans in this book aren't just theoretical recommendations; they are practices that have been lived, felt, and benefited from by people like you and me.

My experience with Wall Pilates isn't just academic; it's personal. It has transformed not just my body, but my sense of self. I'm not just the author of this book; I'm a living testament to its potential. I wrote this guide because I've felt your challenges, lived your questions, and celebrated the same victories you're about to experience. I understand you not because I've read about you, but because I am you.

Are you ready to transform your life, one exercise and one meal at a time? If you've ever felt overlooked by the fitness world, if you've struggled to find routines that understand your body's unique needs as a woman over 40 or a senior, then this book is your key to unlock a new level of health and happiness. I invite you to join me on this 21-day journey of Wall Pilates integrated with a specialized nutrition plan. Don't just read act, because your future self will thank you for taking the step today that will elevate all your tomorrows. Let's turn the page and start this exciting chapter of renewed vitality together—your transformation starts now!

Chapter 1
Wall Pilates 101

Pilates, a practice often viewed as a floor activity, possesses a transformative quality when combined with a simple wall. The wall, a steadfast support in our homes, becomes an anchor in Wall Pilates, offering both challenge and security. As we begin to explore the essentials of this practice, the wall becomes more than just support; it becomes an active participant in our fitness routine, providing resistance, feedback, and structure.

To truly benefit from Wall Pilates, we must first understand its core principles. These principles don't just guide our physical movements but also shape our mindset. Each one encourages us to achieve greater balance, strength, and well-being. By truly embracing them, we create a foundation for a healthier life.

Before we dive into specific exercises and techniques, let's first familiarize ourselves with these guiding principles. Their significance cannot be understated, as they shape each movement, ensuring it's safe, effective, and beneficial.

These principles — breathing, centering, control, precision, flow, and the power of the mind — act as pillars, ensuring every session leaves us feeling rejuvenated and stronger. By the end of this chapter, you'll have a firm grasp of what Wall Pilates can offer and how it differs from traditional Pilates.

With a wall by your side, you're not just taking on a new set of exercises; you're adopting a fresh perspective on fitness. One where every push, pull, and stretch brings a new chance to strengthen, balance, and rejuvenate. Whether you're a seasoned Pilates enthusiast or new to the practice, Wall Pilates promises a refreshing twist to the beloved routine. So, let's start this exploration together and discover the wonders of Wall Pilates.

The Art of Breathing Right

Breathing is the most natural act, isn't it? From the moment we come into this world to our last second, breathing remains a constant. It keeps us alive, and sustains us through moments of joy, sadness, and everything in between. However, most of us seldom pay attention to how we breathe, even though it plays a pivotal role in our overall health and well-being.

Wall Pilates, with its focus on physical form and mindful movement, shines a spotlight on the significance of breathing correctly. Breathing, in this practice, isn't just about supplying oxygen to the body; it's a tool, an anchor, that enhances every exercise and makes it more effective.

Imagine a balloon. If you were to inflate it partially and then try to shape it, it would be somewhat pliable but not very responsive. Fill it too much, and it becomes tense, almost bursting. But if you inflate it just right, it achieves an optimal shape and flexibility. Similarly, our lungs and diaphragm operate best when we use them effectively, helping our body maintain an ideal state of relaxation and tension.

So, how does one master the art of breathing right in Wall Pilates?

Understanding the Diaphragm

First, let's talk about the diaphragm. This dome-shaped muscle sits below the lungs and plays a star role in breathing. When it contracts, it moves downward, creating space for the lungs to expand. As it relaxes, it moves up, pushing out the air. It's this simple movement, often overlooked, that holds the key to breathing correctly in Wall Pilates.

Deep Breathing versus Shallow Breathing

Many of us are used to shallow breathing, especially when stressed or in a hurry. It's a rapid inhalation and exhalation, mostly using the chest. This type of breathing doesn't maximize the oxygen intake, leading to decreased energy and focus.

In contrast, deep breathing involves both the diaphragm and the chest. It's a full and rhythmic inhalation followed by a complete exhalation, ensuring that the body gets all the oxygen it needs while expelling waste efficiently.

The Wall Pilates Breathing Technique

In Wall Pilates, breathing turns into an art form. The wall, being our guide, helps us visualize and feel our breaths more distinctly. Here's a basic technique:

- Stand with your back against the wall. Feel the cool, steady presence of the wall behind you.
- Place one hand on your chest and the other on your abdomen.
- Breathe in slowly through your nose, directing the breath towards the abdomen. You should feel the hand on your abdomen rise, while the one on your chest remains relatively still.
- Now, exhale slowly through the mouth, feeling the abdomen fall back.

This exercise demonstrates diaphragmatic breathing, ensuring that you're using the diaphragm effectively. With the wall as support, it becomes easier to focus and understand the movement of breath in and out of the body.

Benefits of Breathing Right in Wall Pilates

1. **Improved Oxygenation**: Proper breathing ensures every cell in the body gets the oxygen it needs. This can lead to increased energy levels and improved cellular function.
2. **Better Muscle Function**: Oxygen is crucial for muscle function. With improved oxygenation, muscles can work more efficiently, reducing the risk of cramps and fatigue.
3. **Enhanced Focus**: When you breathe deeply, you're also supplying more oxygen to the brain. This can sharpen your focus, helping you execute Pilates movements with precision.
4. **Stress Reduction**: Deep breathing activates the body's relaxation response. It can lower stress hormones, slow down the heart rate, and induce a sense of calm.
5. **Stabilized Core**: Breathing engages the core muscles, especially the deep abdominal muscles. When done right, it aids in stabilizing the core, which is essential for most Pilates exercises.

The beauty of Wall Pilates breathing is that it doesn't require any special equipment or setting. You can practice it anytime, anywhere. Over time, this technique will become second nature, enhancing not just your Pilates workouts but also your day-to-day life.

So, while breathing is a natural act, doing it correctly can make a world of difference. In Wall Pilates, the act of breathing transcends its basic function, becoming a bridge between mind and body. When harnessed effectively, it can amplify the benefits of each exercise, leading to improved health, vitality, and a sense of well-being.

Finding Your Center, literally!

In the vast expanse of our bodies, there exists a central point, an anchor, which holds the power to transform our posture, balance, and movement. This central point, often referred to as the 'center' in Pilates, isn't a mystical or abstract idea. It's real, tangible, and plays a vital role in our overall physical well-being.

So, what exactly is this 'center'? And why is it so crucial in Wall Pilates?

The Anatomy of the Center

The center refers to a group of muscles in our body's midsection. This includes the deep abdominal muscles, the muscles around the spine, the pelvic floor, and the diaphragm. Together, they create a corset-like structure, supporting the spine, organs, and the entire upper body.

But here's the thing: many daily activities, from sitting for long hours to lifting heavy objects, can weaken these muscles. Over time, this can lead to poor posture, back pain, and reduced core strength.

Why the Center Matters in Wall Pilates

Wall Pilates offers a unique advantage in locating and strengthening the center. The wall, with its solid and unmoving presence, provides tactile feedback, making it easier to activate and engage the center during exercises.

By focusing on the center, Wall Pilates does more than just sculpt the midsection. It brings about:

1. **Improved Posture**: A strong center provides better support to the spine, promoting a straighter, more aligned posture.
2. **Enhanced Balance**: Balance isn't just about the legs. A firm center offers stability, reducing the chances of falls and wobbles.
3. **Efficient Movement**: Movements powered by a strong center are more fluid and efficient, reducing strain on other muscles.
4. **Protection Against Injuries**: A robust center acts as a shield, absorbing shocks and stresses, and thus minimizing the risk of injuries.

Discovering Your Center with Wall Pilates

Now, the big question: How can one find and strengthen the center using Wall Pilates?

- **Breath Awareness**: As discussed in the previous section, breathing plays a significant role in Pilates. By breathing deeply and fully, you can engage the diaphragm and the deep abdominal muscles, which are core components of the center.
- **Visualization**: Stand with your back against the wall. Picture a line running from the base of your skull, down the spine, and to the tailbone. This line represents your center. As you practice Wall Pilates exercises, imagine this line staying straight and strong.
- **Activate the Core**: Before beginning any exercise, consciously tighten the abdominal muscles. It's not about sucking in the stomach but rather about drawing the belly button gently towards the spine.
- **Feel the Wall**: The wall can be a fantastic guide. As you perform exercises, be mindful of how your body contacts the wall. This feedback can help in ensuring that the center remains engaged and active throughout the routine.

Strengthening the Center - A Daily Commitment

The center's muscles, like any other muscle, need regular exercise to stay strong. While Wall Pilates provides a structured routine to work on the center, it's essential to engage it even outside of exercise sessions. Whether you're walking, sitting, or lifting something, being aware of the center and keeping it activated can go a long way in improving core strength and stability.

In Wall Pilates, the center isn't just a physical point; it represents a balanced and harmonious state where the body and mind come together. By locating and strengthening the center, individuals lay down a solid foundation upon which the rest of the Wall Pilates exercises build. It is this focus on the core, the very essence of our physical being, that sets Wall Pilates apart and makes it such a transformative practice.

With a strong center, individuals not only enhance their Pilates practice but also improve the quality of their daily life, enjoying better posture, fewer aches, and a more active and agile body.

Control: No, We're Not Talking About Remote Controls

In a world where fast and furious seems to be the motto, slowing down and taking charge of our movements might sound counterintuitive. But in the universe of Wall Pilates, control reigns supreme. It's not about speed or showing off complicated moves; it's about mastering the simplicity of each movement with grace and, yes, control.

Control, in this context, isn't about power or dominance. It's about awareness, precision, and intention in every move you make. Think of it this way: if our bodies were vehicles, control would be the fine-tuned steering system guiding us smoothly around life's many corners.

Why Control Matters in Wall Pilates

Wall Pilates is a practice that brings movement and mindfulness together. Every exercise requires a delicate balance of strength and flexibility, of effort and ease. Without control, it's easy to miss the mark, making exercises less effective or even risking injury.

Here are some key reasons why control holds such a prominent place in Wall Pilates:

1. **Safety First**: Controlled movements ensure that you don't push your body beyond its limits. It minimizes the risk of strains, sprains, or any other injuries.

2. **Efficiency is Key**: When you move with control, every muscle works in harmony, making exercises more efficient and effective. You're not just flailing around; you're making every second and every movement count.
3. **Mind-Body Connection**: Control isn't just physical; it's mental too. By focusing on controlled movements, you're also training your mind to be present, attentive, and alert.

The Wall: The Ultimate Tool for Control

The wall is not just a prop; it's a partner in your Pilates practice. It provides feedback, offers resistance, and acts as a guide. When you lean into it or push against it, you can feel the force, the tension, and the alignment of your body. This tactile feedback is invaluable in mastering control.

For example, when practicing a Wall Pilates leg lift, the wall can help you gauge if your hips are aligned, if your back is straight, and if you're lifting your leg with control rather than momentum.

Practicing Control in Wall Pilates

Control is like a muscle; the more you practice, the stronger it gets. Here are some ways to cultivate control in your Wall Pilates routine:

- **Start Slow**: Especially if you're new to Wall Pilates, take it slow. It's not a race. Focus on understanding and mastering the movement rather than rushing through it.
- **Prioritize Quality Over Quantity**: It's better to do five controlled, precise repetitions than fifteen hurried ones. Remember, it's not about how many you do but how well you do them.
- **Stay Connected to Your Breath**: Your breath is a natural metronome. Use it to guide your movements. For example, inhale as you lift your leg, and exhale as you lower it. This breath-movement connection can help ensure controlled and rhythmic exercises.
- **Engage Your Core**: Your center, as discussed earlier, is the powerhouse of your body. By engaging it, you provide stability and support, making controlled movements easier.

- **Use the Wall as Feedback**: Pay attention to how your body feels against the wall. If you're pressing too hard or leaning too much, you'll know. The wall doesn't lie.

The Ripple Effect of Control

Mastering control in Wall Pilates can have a ripple effect on other areas of life. You may find yourself moving with more grace and intention, whether you're lifting groceries, playing with your kids, or dancing the night away. Control, in essence, teaches us to move through life with mindfulness, precision, and a certain elegance.

While the concept of control might sound restrictive or confining, in Wall Pilates, it's quite the opposite. It's liberating. It's the key to unlocking the true potential of each movement, ensuring safety, efficiency, and a deep sense of connection between the mind and body. So, the next time you stand next to that wall, ready to start your exercise, remember to take charge, move with intention, and let the magic of control elevate your Wall Pilates experience.

Precision: It's All in the Details

In the gentle and methodical world of Wall Pilates, there's an underlying principle that enhances every stretch, every bend, and every lift: precision. It isn't about making large, dramatic moves. Instead, it's about the subtle shifts, the tiny adjustments, the minute changes that make all the difference.

Think of a sculptor, chiseling away at a block of marble. It isn't the forceful blows that reveal the statue within, but the careful, deliberate chipping away, piece by piece. Similarly, in Wall Pilates, precision turns every movement into a work of art, where the details hold the key to transformation.

Why Precision is Paramount in Wall Pilates

Precision in Wall Pilates isn't just for the sake of aesthetics or perfection. It serves a multitude of purposes:

1. **Safety**: Accurate movements mean you're less likely to overextend a muscle or strain a joint. Precision ensures that every movement is aligned, balanced, and safe.
2. **Effectiveness**: The difference between a good exercise and a great one often lies in the details. By being precise, you ensure that the targeted muscles are engaged and worked upon optimally.
3. **Building Body Awareness**: Precision demands attention. As you focus on the details of each movement, you become more attuned to your body, understanding its strengths, limitations, and nuances.

The Role of the Wall in Cultivating Precision

The wall isn't just a surface; it's a feedback mechanism. Its steadfast nature provides instant feedback, letting you know if you're leaning too much to one side, if your hips are tilted, or if your shoulders are uneven. This immediate feedback loop helps refine movements, ensuring that every exercise is done with the utmost precision.

Steps to Achieve Precision in Wall Pilates

- **Educate Yourself**: Before diving into an exercise, understand its purpose. Knowing which muscles you're targeting or what you're aiming to achieve can guide your movements.
- **Stay Mindful**: Be present in the moment. Instead of rushing through a routine, take your time. Feel each stretch, each contraction. Listen to your body.
- **Use Mirrors**: A mirror can be a helpful tool. It offers a visual cue, allowing you to see if you're aligned correctly or if you need to make adjustments.
- **Consistency is Key**: Precision is honed over time. The more you practice, the more precise your movements will become. Over time, what seems like a tiny, almost insignificant adjustment can lead to noticeable improvements in strength, flexibility, and posture.
- **Seek Feedback**: If possible, practice Wall Pilates with a buddy or under the guidance of a trained instructor. Sometimes, an external perspective can catch details you might miss.

Precision Beyond the Wall

The beauty of precision, as practiced in Wall Pilates, is that its benefits extend beyond the mat. As you cultivate precision in your exercises, you may notice its positive effects in other areas of your life. Whether it's the way you sit at your desk, how you walk, or even in tasks that require fine motor skills, a precise approach can lead to better outcomes and reduced strain.

To sum it up, precision in Wall Pilates isn't about perfectionism. It's about understanding that every detail, no matter how small, plays a part in the larger picture. It's about recognizing that sometimes, less is more. A slight tilt of the pelvis, a gentle flex of the foot, or a subtle shift in weight can elevate an exercise from good to great.

As you continue your Wall Pilates practice, embrace precision as a trusted companion. Let it guide your movements, refine your techniques, and elevate your practice. After all, in the world of Wall Pilates, it truly is all in the details.

Chapter 2
Understanding Pilates and its Origins

The world of fitness and health is vast, offering countless ways for people to strengthen their bodies, boost flexibility, and enhance overall well-being. Among these, Pilates stands out as a unique method that has stood the test of time, proving its value to countless individuals. To appreciate the depth of this method, one must first understand its roots and foundational principles. This chapter will guide you through the fascinating history of Pilates, its core principles, and how the concept of wall Pilates emerged as a practical adaptation for diverse groups like women and seniors.

The History of Pilates

In the early 20th century, a new approach to body conditioning and rehabilitation began to take shape, offering a unique blend of strength, flexibility, and mindfulness. This method, known today as Pilates, emerged from the creativity and determination of one man: Joseph Pilates.

Born in Germany in 1883, Joseph battled various ailments as a child, from asthma to rickets. These early health challenges fueled his passion for physical fitness. He became involved in multiple athletic pursuits, from gymnastics and skiing to boxing and diving. The combination of these activities offered him insights into how the body moved, functioned, and healed.

Joseph's initial system was aptly named "Contrology". The focus was on the art of controlled movements. In his view, physical health and mental well-being were deeply intertwined. To him, the ultimate goal wasn't just muscular strength but a harmonious balance between body and mind.

World events played a significant role in the development and spread of Joseph's methodology. During World War I, he found himself in an internment camp in England because of his German citizenship. But adversity often breeds innovation. While at the camp, Joseph started developing his exercise regimen further, assisting fellow internees in regaining strength and overcoming injuries. This environment became a testing ground for his methods.

In the confines of the camp, he devised equipment prototypes using the limited materials available, like bed springs. These initial prototypes later inspired some of the classic Pilates equipment we know today, such as the Reformer.

After the war, Joseph returned to Germany and continued to refine his methods, working closely with dancers, athletes, and other experts. However, as the political climate in Germany became more turbulent in the 1920s, Joseph decided to leave. He chose New York City as his new home.

Once in New York, Joseph and his wife, Clara, opened a fitness studio. The location was strategic; it was close to many dance studios and theaters. As a result, many dancers, who were always on the lookout for effective ways to improve strength and recover from injuries, found their way to Pilates. They became some of the earliest and most enthusiastic adopters of the method. Names like George Balanchine and Martha Graham, pillars of the dance world, became proponents of Joseph's methods.

The exercises focused on core strength, flexibility, and balance. The emphasis was on quality over quantity and precision over repetition. Every movement had a purpose, and the focus was on doing each exercise with utmost care and attention to detail.

While Joseph's methods gained popularity, it was the trainees and disciples who played a pivotal role in ensuring its longevity. As they learned from the master, they added their own insights and adaptations. Over time, these students opened their own studios, ensuring the teachings of Joseph spread far and wide.

One of the most notable students was Romana Kryzanowska. She not only mastered the art but took it upon herself to train future instructors, ensuring the legacy continued in its purest form. She became a beacon of Pilates, maintaining its essence while allowing for its evolution.

Over the decades, Pilates has seen various adaptations and evolutions. From mat-based exercises to complex equipment, the core essence of mindful movement remains unchanged. Today, millions across the globe practice Pilates, a testament to its effectiveness and the vision of its creator.

As time passed, innovations like wall Pilates emerged. These adaptations allowed for a broader range of people, including women and seniors, to benefit from the practice. Tailoring exercises to individual needs, focusing on safety, and ensuring accessibility became pivotal in these new approaches.

In summary, the history of Pilates is a testament to the passion and perseverance of one man who believed in the power of controlled movement. From its humble beginnings in an internment camp to its global recognition, Pilates remains a favored method for those seeking a balanced approach to fitness. The blend of strength, flexibility, and mindfulness it offers is as relevant today as it was a century ago.

Key Principles of Pilates

Behind every method that stands the test of time, there is a foundation of solid principles. These guiding lights ensure that even as the method adapts and grows, its core remains unshaken. For Pilates, these principles are more than just guidelines; they are the essence of the practice, ensuring it delivers on its promise of balanced body conditioning.

CenteringPilates often speaks of the "powerhouse" of the body. This isn't a reference to sheer muscular strength but rather a focal point from which all energy for exercise emanates. Located roughly in the center of the body, encompassing the abdomen, lower back, hips, and buttocks, this central hub is where all Pilates movements should begin. By emphasizing this core strength, Pilates aids in developing a strong, stable foundation for every action, whether in a Pilates class or in daily life.

Concentration

Mindfulness might seem like a modern trend, but Pilates had it figured out long ago. The emphasis in Pilates isn't on mindlessly repeating movements but on performing each exercise with full attention. By focusing intently on each movement, practitioners can achieve the maximum benefit from each exercise and ensure it's done correctly, reducing the risk of injury.

Control

There's no room for wild, uncontrolled movements in Pilates. Instead, every motion is deliberate. This isn't about restriction but about mastery. Control in Pilates means understanding how the body works and moving it with precision. Such mastery ensures that every muscle is engaged appropriately, making the exercise regimen effective and efficient.

Breathing

To breathe might seem the most natural thing in the world, but Pilates brings it to the forefront of consciousness. The method emphasizes full, deep inhalations and exhalations. The act of breathing in Pilates is structured to oxygenate the blood, which then stimulates the brain and revitalizes the body. More than that, controlled breathing helps in flushing out toxins and supports better posture and muscle activation. By syncing specific movements with breath patterns, Pilates ensures a harmonious rhythm in workouts, providing both mental clarity and physical vitality.

Flow

Fluidity is at the heart of Pilates. Each exercise seamlessly transitions into the next, ensuring a graceful flow throughout the session. This principle is not just about aesthetics or smoothness. It's about efficiency and function. A continuous, flowing movement through the exercise sequence boosts muscular endurance and improves strength without putting undue strain on the body.

Precision

Quality over quantity is a mantra that resonates deeply within the Pilates practice. Instead of focusing on countless repetitions, the emphasis is on doing each exercise with exact precision. This meticulous approach ensures that the right muscles are engaged, fostering better results in less time. It's not about how many times a movement is performed but about how well it's executed.

Alignment

Posture and proper alignment are paramount in Pilates. The method places a strong emphasis on maintaining a neutral spine and correct skeletal alignment throughout every exercise. By doing so, it ensures that the body is balanced and that stress is distributed evenly across muscles and joints. This emphasis not only prevents injuries but also promotes a better posture outside of the Pilates sessions.

In understanding these key principles, the beauty of Pilates becomes evident. It's more than just a series of exercises; it's a holistic approach to body and mind wellness. The principles aren't rigid rules but guiding stars, helping practitioners navigate their workouts with purpose and awareness.

But why are these principles so vital? The genius of Pilates lies in its integration of these concepts. Each one supports the other, creating a harmonized system where the whole is indeed greater than the sum of its parts. By centering the body, focusing the mind, controlling movements, breathing deeply, moving with the flow, acting with precision, and maintaining alignment, one is not just exercising; they're engaging in a fully integrated body conditioning system.

The universality of these principles also ensures that Pilates is adaptable. Whether it's the classic mat workouts or the innovative wall Pilates, these core tenets remain the same, ensuring consistent benefits regardless of specific routines or equipment.

In the panorama of fitness methods, Pilates stands out, not just for its effectiveness but for its deep-rooted philosophy. The principles lay a strong foundation, ensuring that as the world changes and as people's needs evolve, Pilates remains a constant beacon of balanced fitness, offering strength, flexibility, and peace of mind to those who embrace its teachings.

The Evolution of Wall Pilates

The world of fitness is never static. Over time, as people's needs change and our understanding of the human body grows, methods evolve. Such has been the case with Pilates. From its early days under Joseph Pilates' guidance to the diverse styles we see today, Pilates has consistently adapted while maintaining its core principles. Among the many adaptations, one stands out for its accessibility and practicality: Wall Pilates.

To trace the origins of Wall Pilates, it's essential to consider the broader context of fitness evolution. In the late 20th century, a trend began where fitness experts and enthusiasts started looking for ways to make exercise regimes more accessible. There was a growing recognition that not everyone had access to specialized equipment or the capability to perform floor exercises.

Around this time, some innovative Pilates instructors began to experiment. They sought to bring the benefits of traditional Pilates to a wider audience, especially those who might find mat exercises challenging. Whether it was due to age, injury, or just personal preference, there was a clear need for alternatives.

This led to the birth of Wall Pilates. Using the wall as a supportive tool, instructors developed exercises that mirrored many of the traditional Pilates moves but with the added stability the wall provided. Instead of relying on gravity as in mat Pilates, Wall Pilates leverages the vertical plane, providing a different kind of resistance and support.

The benefits were immediately apparent. First and foremost, the wall provided stability, reducing the risk of falls and making it especially beneficial for seniors or those with balance issues. For beginners or those recovering from injuries, the wall offered a gentle way to build strength and flexibility without the risk of overexertion.

Additionally, Wall Pilates also introduced a new range of motion and exercises. The vertical plane allowed for movements that weren't possible on a mat. This added diversity made workouts more engaging and opened up a new set of challenges even for seasoned Pilates enthusiasts.

However, the true beauty of Wall Pilates lay in its simplicity. No elaborate equipment was needed; a flat wall was sufficient. This simplicity made it perfect for home workouts, a feature that gained importance in the 21st century as more and more people looked for effective home-based exercise regimes.

Over the years, Wall Pilates has grown in popularity. Numerous studios around the world offer specialized classes, and there's no shortage of online resources for those who prefer to practice at home. Many instructors have further innovated, incorporating props like resistance bands or softballs to add variety to the workouts.

While Wall Pilates is an evolution of the traditional method, it remains faithful to the core principles. Centering, concentration, control, breathing, flow, precision, and alignment are all integral to the practice, ensuring its effectiveness.

In many ways, Wall Pilates reflects the enduring spirit of Joseph Pilates' original vision. It's a testament to the method's adaptability and relevance. By offering a blend of challenge and accessibility, Wall Pilates ensures that the benefits of this unique exercise system are available to an even broader audience.

To conclude, Wall Pilates is not just an offshoot; it's a significant chapter in the ongoing story of Pilates. It represents the method's ability to grow, adapt, and meet the needs of people in changing times. With its unique set of exercises and emphasis on accessibility, Wall Pilates has firmly established itself as a vital part of the Pilates family, bringing strength, flexibility, and balance to countless individuals around the world.

Chapter 3
The Science Behind Wall Pilates

Wall Pilates emerges as a beacon of simplicity, yet its effects are profound. Rooted in science, this method offers a unique blend of strength, flexibility, and control. The wall, a humble barrier we often overlook, transforms into a tool of wellness and vitality under the guidance of Wall Pilates.

This technique rests on scientific principles that harness the body's natural movements and potentials. While many may view a wall as just a boundary, Wall Pilates sees it as an ally. It aids in enhancing our posture, improving muscle tone, and refining our sense of balance. As we press against it, the wall offers resistance, making our muscles work harder, yet in a controlled manner. This resistance acts as a guide, ensuring that exercises are done accurately, optimizing benefits, and minimizing risks.

As we explore further, we'll uncover the myriad of benefits Wall Pilates brings to different groups. For women, it can be a game changer in addressing specific needs, from enhancing core strength to fostering better posture. For our senior community, Wall Pilates can be a gentle yet effective way to maintain muscle tone, flexibility, and overall mobility. And for everyone, the emphasis on balance and stability holds the promise of a life where each step is confident and sure.

As you read on, you'll discover the detailed advantages of this method. By understanding the science and logic behind Wall Pilates, you'll be better equipped to appreciate its value and perhaps, make it a part of your fitness routine. So, let's dive deeper into the benefits of Wall Pilates for different groups, starting with its significance for women.

Benefits for Women

Wall Pilates, a unique twist in the fitness spectrum, has swiftly gained attention for its distinctive approach. With its foundation rooted in time-tested principles of exercise and physiology, Wall Pilates offers an array of benefits tailor-made for women of all ages.

At the heart of this technique is the unassuming wall. More than just a vertical surface, the wall in Wall Pilates is a partner, a guide, and a force that amplifies the impact of each movement. While its merits are vast, let's focus on what it brings to the table specifically for women.

Strength and Toning

A common goal among many women is to achieve toned muscles without the bulkiness. Wall Pilates stands out in this regard. The exercises designed around this method concentrate on using the body's own weight and the resistance provided by the wall. This approach leads to the development of lean muscle mass. Over time, regular practice can result in sculpted arms, defined legs, and a strong core.

Flexibility

As women age, flexibility can decline, leading to stiffness and discomfort. Wall Pilates offers a gentle way to stretch and lengthen muscles. The wall acts as a support, allowing for deeper stretches while ensuring safety. Regular participation can lead to enhanced flexibility, leading to a more fluid range of motion and decreased risk of injuries.

Bone Density

Osteoporosis is a concern for many women, especially post-menopause. Engaging in weight-bearing exercises is one of the recommended ways to combat bone density loss. Wall Pilates, with its emphasis on resistance and weight-bearing movements, can be beneficial in this aspect. The act of pushing against the wall and holding certain postures can aid in maintaining and even improving bone health.

Core Development

The core, a group of muscles enveloping our midsection, plays a pivotal role in our overall health and function. A strong core supports the spine, ensures good posture, and aids in daily activities. Wall Pilates focuses heavily on core engagement. The exercises often involve holding postures against the wall, which demands core activation. Over time, this leads to a stronger, more defined midsection, which is not only aesthetically pleasing but also crucial for spinal health.

Stress Relief

Modern life, with its whirlwind of responsibilities, can be taxing. Finding an outlet to release stress becomes essential for mental well-being. Wall Pilates, with its emphasis on controlled breathing and mindful movement, becomes more than just a physical workout. The rhythmic breathing patterns, coupled with the gentle flow of exercises, can induce a state of calm and relaxation. For women juggling multiple roles, this can be a sanctuary, a time to reconnect with oneself and find a moment of peace amidst the chaos.

Postnatal Recovery

Childbirth, a transformative event, brings along physical changes. Postnatal recovery is a phase where many women seek safe and effective ways to regain their pre-pregnancy form and function. Wall Pilates, with its gentle nature, can be an excellent choice. The exercises can be modified to cater to postnatal needs, focusing on strengthening the pelvic floor, toning the abdominal muscles, and improving overall stamina.

Hormonal Balance

Exercise, in general, has been shown to have a positive impact on hormonal health. Wall Pilates, with its combination of strength, flexibility, and relaxation exercises, can aid in balancing hormones. Regular practice can lead to better regulation of hormones such as cortisol, the stress hormone, and endorphins, the feel-good hormones. This can result in improved mood, better sleep, and enhanced overall well-being.

Wall Pilates, with its simple yet effective approach, brings a bouquet of benefits tailored for women. Whether one seeks physical strength, mental relaxation, or hormonal balance, this method offers solutions. Its beauty lies in its adaptability. It can be molded to fit the needs of women across different life stages, from youth to senior years. As we move forward, it's essential to recognize and embrace the potential of Wall Pilates, not just as a fitness regimen, but as a holistic approach to women's well-being.

Benefits for Seniors

Wall Pilates, with its unique approach to fitness, has opened doors to a world of well-being for many, especially seniors. The simplicity of using a wall as the primary tool bridges the gap between challenging workouts and accessible exercises. Let's explore how this fitness method caters to the senior population, offering benefits that resonate with their specific needs.

Safety First

One of the main concerns for seniors when it comes to exercise is safety. The fear of falls or injuries can be a deterrent. Wall Pilates addresses this concern head-on. The wall acts as a sturdy support, allowing seniors to perform exercises with added confidence. This stable backing reduces the risk of falls and ensures that movements are controlled and precise.

Joint Health

Age often brings about stiffness in the joints. Movements become less fluid, and discomfort can become a daily companion. Wall Pilates offers exercises that encourage a range of motion. These movements, though gentle, can help in lubricating the joints, reducing stiffness, and increasing mobility. Over time, seniors might find tasks like bending, turning, or even simple walking becoming easier.

Muscle Maintenance

Muscle mass tends to decrease with age. This decline can lead to weakness and reduced stamina. Wall Pilates emphasizes resistance training. Pushing against the wall, holding postures, and performing controlled movements can aid in maintaining, if not improving, muscle strength. Regular practice can result in stronger arms, legs, and core, making daily activities less strenuous.

Improved Posture

Aging can bring about postural changes. Many seniors develop a forward head posture or a rounded back. Wall Pilates focuses heavily on spinal alignment. The exercises encourage upright postures, and the wall acts as a constant reminder to keep the spine straight. Over time, this can lead to improved posture, reducing the strain on the spine and associated discomfort.

Balance and Coordination

Balance is a crucial aspect of daily life, more so for seniors. A minor imbalance can lead to falls, which can have serious repercussions in the golden years. Wall Pilates, with its emphasis on stability exercises, can enhance balance. The wall, ever-present, offers support, allowing seniors to challenge their balance in a safe environment. Coupled with coordination exercises, Wall Pilates can be a comprehensive solution to improve overall stability.

Mental Well-being

Exercise isn't just about physical health. The mental benefits are just as vital, especially for seniors who might be dealing with loneliness, anxiety, or cognitive decline. Wall Pilates, with its combination of movement and breathing, can act as a form of meditation. The rhythmic nature of exercises can lead to a calm mind, reduced anxiety, and even improved cognitive function. The act of focusing on postures, breathing patterns, and movement sequences can enhance concentration and mental clarity.

Social Interaction

While Wall Pilates can be practiced alone, joining a group class can offer the added benefit of social interaction. Meeting peers, sharing experiences, and enjoying a communal activity can be uplifting. In an age where isolation can be a concern, Wall Pilates offers an avenue for seniors to connect, share, and grow together.

Flexibility

While it might seem that flexibility is a trait of the young, it's never too late to work on it. Wall Pilates, with its series of stretches and lengthening exercises, can lead to improved flexibility even in the senior years. The wall acts as a support, allowing for deeper, safer stretches. With consistent practice, seniors might find an increased range of motion, making movements smoother and more comfortable.

Age is just a number, but the challenges it brings can sometimes be overwhelming. Wall Pilates offers a beacon of hope, a path that ensures that the golden years are not just about slowing down but thriving with grace. The benefits it brings to the table for seniors are vast and significant. From physical strength to mental peace, from improved balance to social connections, Wall Pilates is more than just a fitness method; it's a way of life, ensuring that the senior years are filled with vitality, joy, and well-being.

Improving Balance and Stability

Balance and stability, fundamental to our daily activities, become more than just physical attributes; they are anchors that allow us to move with confidence and grace. Wall Pilates, with its unique approach, offers a promising route to enhance these essential aspects of our physical well-being.

The Foundation of Balance

Before diving into the benefits and techniques, it's essential to understand what balance really means. At its core, balance is the ability to maintain our body's center of mass over its base of support. It's what allows us to stand on one foot, walk on uneven surfaces, or even sit without toppling over. Multiple systems work in tandem to ensure we stay balanced, including our visual system, vestibular system (inner ear), and proprioception (sensing the position of our limbs).

Wall Pilates and Its Emphasis on Stability

Wall Pilates uniquely integrates the use of a wall as a supportive tool. This straightforward addition transforms traditional exercises by providing a constant point of reference. The wall not only acts as a support but also gives immediate feedback. If one leans too much to one side or doesn't align correctly, the wall is there to signal the discrepancy.

Techniques to Boost Balance

Wall Pilates incorporates various exercises that challenge and enhance balance. Some of these include single-leg stands, where one foot is placed against the wall while standing on the other, or wall planks, where hands are pressed against the wall, and the body is held in a straight line.

But what makes these exercises truly effective is the combination of movement and resistance. By pushing against the wall or trying to maintain a posture with the wall's assistance, one engages multiple muscle groups. This not only strengthens the muscles but also improves the neuromuscular coordination necessary for balance.

Stability: More than Just Strength

While strength is a component of stability, there's more to the story. Stability involves the ability to control movement, especially when faced with external forces or disturbances. Wall Pilates, with its emphasis on controlled, deliberate movements, fosters this control. Exercises often involve slow, measured motions against the wall's resistance, training the body to move with intention and precision.

Benefits Beyond the Physical

While the primary goal might be to improve physical balance and stability, Wall Pilates offers more. The act of focusing on posture, alignment, and controlled movements has a meditative quality. This focus not only calms the mind but also enhances body awareness. Over time, one becomes more attuned to their body's position in space, its alignment, and its movements, further aiding in balance and stability.

Adaptable for All Levels

One of the standout features of Wall Pilates is its adaptability. Whether one is a beginner or has been practicing for years, exercises can be modified to suit individual needs. For those just starting out or facing significant balance challenges, the wall offers full support. As one progresses, the reliance on the wall can be reduced, increasing the challenge and further enhancing balance and stability.

Practical Implications

Improved balance and stability have real-world implications. From preventing falls to making daily tasks easier, the benefits seep into everyday life. Walking becomes steadier, standing in queues less tiresome, and even activities like climbing stairs or carrying groceries become more manageable. In essence, Wall Pilates doesn't just enhance balance and stability; it improves the quality of life.

In a world where fast and intense often becomes the mantra for fitness, Wall Pilates stands as a testament to the power of simplicity. Improving balance and stability might not sound as glamorous as building muscle or shedding pounds, but their impact on daily life is undeniable. Through controlled movements, resistance training, and a focus on body awareness, Wall Pilates offers a holistic approach to these vital aspects of physical well-being. By integrating this method into one's routine, the promise isn't just of better balance but of a life lived with more confidence, grace, and poise.

Chapter 4
Getting Started with Wall Pilates

When we think of Pilates, most of us imagine large equipment or mats spread out on the floor. But wall Pilates? Now that might sound a little different, right? Yet, the beauty of wall Pilates lies in its simplicity and effectiveness. With the support of a sturdy wall, many exercises become accessible, even to those who might have thought Pilates was out of reach for them. Especially for our focused audience of women and seniors, the wall becomes a dependable partner in these exercises, offering support and stability.

For many, the wall offers a sense of safety. It's steadfast, unwavering, and always there to lean on—literally! With wall Pilates, we utilize this reliable support to enhance our workouts and get the most out of each movement. You don't need a lot to start; in fact, the wall and your own body are the primary tools. But, as with any exercise routine, a few basic preparations can help ensure you get the most benefit and enjoyment out of your sessions.

Necessary Equipment and Setup

Ah, the thrill of starting something new. It can be akin to setting up a new space in the home or organizing a room. Wall Pilates, a wonderfully effective and accessible form of exercise, doesn't ask for much. But for those who prefer a touch of preparation to ensure they're all set; this section is dedicated to helping create the perfect environment for effective wall Pilates sessions.

Let's begin by clarifying a fundamental point: wall Pilates is incredibly simple. The primary "equipment" you need is a wall. Yet, for those keen on perfecting their space, there are some pieces of equipment and setup tips that can amplify the experience.

Choosing the Right Wall

A wall might seem like just another part of the house, but for wall Pilates, it becomes an essential part of the routine. The first step is to find a clear wall space. This means a wall without paintings, decorations, or other obstructions that might hinder movement. The wall surface should be smooth to prevent scratches or discomfort. Also, ensure it's sturdy and free from any damage.

Floor Matters

The ground you stand on while performing wall Pilates is equally significant. A non-slip floor is essential. Wooden or tiled floors can sometimes be slippery, especially if you're wearing socks. Consider using a non-slip mat or going barefoot to ensure a good grip. Clean the floor of any dust or debris; even a small pebble can throw you off balance.

Comfortable Clothing

Wearing the right clothes can set the tone for your exercise session. Opt for comfortable, stretchy outfits that allow for easy movement. Tight or restrictive clothing can be a hindrance, while loose-fitting clothes can get in the way. Find a balance with clothing that's snug yet flexible.

Optional Tools: The Magic of Small Accessories

While wall Pilates primarily requires just a wall, there are a few accessories that can make certain exercises more comfortable or challenging.

1. **Resistance Bands**: These stretchy bands can be anchored around door handles or heavy furniture close to your wall. They add an element of resistance to certain exercises, intensifying them.
2. **Small Pilates Ball**: This is a soft, inflatable ball, often used to enhance certain wall exercises, especially those targeting the core and inner thighs.
3. **Foam Rollers**: These cylindrical tools can be placed between the wall and your body during specific exercises. They're great for massage, muscle release, and adding variation to the exercises.

4. **Pilates Rings**: Also known as "magic circles," these rings can be used in conjunction with wall exercises to add resistance and target specific muscle groups.

Safety First: Wall Padding

Though not essential, some might prefer adding a layer of padding to their chosen wall, especially if they have sensitive backs or worry about applying too much pressure. Simple yoga mats can be fixed to the wall using removable adhesive hooks. They not only provide cushioning but also add a layer of grip.

A Mirror for Reflection

While the primary goal of wall Pilates is to feel the movements and listen to one's body, having a mirror nearby can be helpful. It allows you to check your form and alignment. However, it's not about striving for perfection; it's about understanding and adapting the exercises to best suit your body.

Setting the Mood: Ambiance and Environment

The environment plays a subtle yet impactful role in any exercise regime. Soft lighting, whether natural or from lamps, can create a peaceful ambiance. Calm and gentle music can soothe the mind and help in focusing on the exercises. Fresh air is also a boon; if possible, choose a spot near a window or ensure the room is well-ventilated.

Keeping Essentials Close

Having a small table or shelf nearby is practical. You can keep water, a towel, or any other essentials you might need. This way, you don't have to disrupt your session by leaving the room.

Safety Precautions and Preparations

Wall Pilates offers a world of benefits, from enhancing strength to increasing flexibility. However, as with any physical activity, moving with mindfulness and understanding some basic precautions can make all the difference between a productive session and an unfortunate mishap.

A Solid Foundation: The Importance of Good Posture

Starting with a neutral posture is a cornerstone of any Pilates practice. But what does this mean? In simple terms, a neutral posture means that the natural curves of the spine are maintained. When standing, the head should align with the shoulders, the shoulders with the hips, and the hips with the ankles. The feet should be hip-width apart, providing a steady base. While the wall is there for support, ensuring your body is well-aligned minimizes the risk of strains.

Warm-Ups: A Gentle Start

Though Wall Pilates is gentle by nature, it's wise to prepare the body with a few warm-up exercises. Simple movements such as shoulder rolls, ankle circles, and gentle side-to-side twists can make the muscles more pliable and responsive. This step is not about intensity; it's about letting the body know that it's time to move.

Watch Those Wrists

Many wall exercises, especially those that involve pushing against the wall, put pressure on the wrists. It's essential to spread the fingers wide and distribute the weight evenly across the palms. If any discomfort is felt in the wrists, it's a sign to adjust the hand position or take a short break.

Mind the Neck

The neck, a delicate part of our anatomy, needs care. Ensure that the neck remains an extension of the spine. Avoid letting the head drop forward or jutting the chin out. For exercises that require looking up or down, move from the upper spine rather than compressing the neck.

The Role of Breathing

Breathing might seem automatic, but in Pilates, it's an integral part of every movement. Breathing deeply and consistently ensures that muscles receive the oxygen they need. It also helps in maintaining focus and rhythm during exercises.

Listening to the Body's Signals

The body communicates constantly, giving signals when things feel right and when they don't. If any sharp pain, dizziness, or discomfort arises, it's essential to stop and assess. It could be a sign that the body needs a different approach or that it's time to rest.

Footwear Considerations

While many prefer to do wall Pilates barefoot for better grip and proprioception, others might opt for footwear. If choosing to wear shoes, they should be comfortable and provide a good grip. Slippery shoes or socks can be a hazard.

Space Aroun

While the main prop is the wall, ensuring there's some free space around is crucial. This allows for unobstructed movement, especially for exercises that involve leg sweeps or arm extensions. A clear area ensures safety and freedom of movement.

Hydration Matters

It might not seem like it, but even low-intensity exercises can lead to dehydration. Keeping a water bottle nearby encourages regular sips, keeping the body hydrated and muscles functioning optimally.

Know the Exit Strategy

This might sound dramatic, but it's practical. For exercises that involve a certain level of balance or leaning against the wall, it's good to know how to safely come out of the position. A controlled exit reduces the risk of sudden strains or falls.

Regular Breaks

Especially for those new to wall Pilates, taking short breaks between exercises can be beneficial. It provides the body a moment to relax, and it's also an opportunity to reset posture and alignment.

End with a Cool Down

Just as the body was warmed up at the start, a cool down at the end helps in gradually bringing the heart rate down and giving the muscles a gentle stretch. Simple stretches targeting the major muscle groups used during the session can aid in recovery and reduce the chances of soreness.

Wall Pilates, with its simplicity and effectiveness, promises a world of benefits. But the true magic lies in blending this effectiveness with safety. Precautions might seem like minor details in the grand scheme, but they play a pivotal role in ensuring each session is not only productive but also safe. With these precautions in mind, one can confidently approach each session, knowing they are giving their body the best of both worlds: strength and safety. So, with a clear wall and these safety tips as companions, the stage is set for an enriching Pilates experience.

Understanding Your Body's Limitations

Every person is a unique blend of strengths, challenges, experiences, and histories. Each body tells a story, marked by the days it danced in the rain, the times it pushed through a fever, the mornings it felt invincible, and the nights it needed some extra care. Wall Pilates, with its accessible charm, welcomes everyone. But to truly harness its potential, it's vital to recognize and respect the boundaries each body sets.

The Importance of Self-awareness

Being aware is the first step in understanding limitations. It's not about drawing a line between what's possible and what's not, but rather, it's about recognizing how the body feels on any given day. There might be days of boundless energy, and then there might be days when even the simplest movement feels challenging.

Past Injuries and Conditions

Past injuries, whether a sprained ankle from a decade ago or a recent muscle strain, play a role in current physical capacities. Old injuries can sometimes lead to protective mechanisms, like favoring one leg over the other. It's essential to be aware of these patterns to ensure they don't interfere with the exercises.

Similarly, medical conditions such as arthritis, osteoporosis, or even heart conditions can influence the body's capabilities. While wall Pilates offers numerous benefits, being mindful of any medical advice or restrictions is crucial.

Flexibility Varies

Flexibility isn't a constant. It can vary based on various factors: the time of day, the weather, or even mood. Pushing the body to stretch beyond its comfort can lead to strains. The goal isn't to mimic a picture-perfect pose but to feel the stretch and benefit from it.

Strength Isn't Just Physical

Physical strength is often the most discussed, but emotional and mental strengths are equally significant. Understanding one's mental state before starting a session can offer insights. If the mind is distracted or stressed, the body might not respond as expected. Being gentle and understanding with oneself on such days can make a difference.

Rest and Recovery

Every body has its own recovery rhythm. For some, after a session of wall Pilates, they might feel ready to conquer the world, while others might need a day of rest. Tuning into these signals is an essential aspect of understanding limitations.

Feedback is Gold

The body constantly gives feedback. A stretch that feels good, a movement that causes discomfort, or even the subtle signs of fatigue are all valuable pieces of information. Treasuring this feedback and adapting accordingly is a key aspect of safe and effective practice.

Consultation and Guidance

If ever in doubt about a particular movement or feeling, consulting a professional can be beneficial. Whether it's a Pilates instructor, a physical therapist, or a medical doctor, their insights can provide clarity and direction.

Adaptation is the Name of the Game

Every exercise in wall Pilates can be adapted to suit individual needs. If a certain movement feels too challenging, there are always modifications to make it more accessible. The beauty of Pilates lies in its adaptability, ensuring everyone, regardless of their limitations, can benefit.

Setting Personal Benchmarks

Instead of comparing oneself with others, setting personal benchmarks can be more rewarding. Maybe today it's about holding a pose for ten seconds, and in a week, it might be fifteen. Celebrating these personal milestones can lead to a deeper appreciation of one's body and its capabilities.

Understanding the body's limitations isn't about setting restrictions. It's about embracing the unique blend that each individual is. It's about dancing to one's own rhythm, even if it's different every day. Wall Pilates, with its promise of strength, flexibility, and balance, becomes a delightful experience when approached with this understanding. It's an invitation to celebrate the body, with all its stories, strengths, and yes, its limitations too.

Chapter 5
Why Women Should Jump on the Wall Pilates Bandwagon

For women, in particular, this form of exercise presents benefits that extend far beyond just a toned physique. Think about the silent battle's women face. The invisible weight of daily responsibilities, the physical transformations from pregnancy, or the natural ebb and flow of aging. While these are all integral parts of a woman's life, they demand a physical and emotional toll. Wall Pilates is not just another item on the list of fitness trends; it's a tool tailored to meet the unique needs of women.

This chapter delves deep into the core reasons why wall Pilates holds a special place in women's fitness. From strengthening the skeletal structure to offering a solution for the much-dreaded mommy tummy, wall Pilates seems to have an answer for it all. For expectant mothers, this exercise promises a partnership that paves the way for a smoother pregnancy. And as the golden years approach, introducing challenges like menopause, wall Pilates stands as a reliable companion, ensuring that the transition is as graceful as possible.

Fortifying Those Bones!

Bones are the very foundation of our bodies, akin to the beams and pillars that hold up a building. They offer support, protect our vital organs, and work hand in hand with our muscles to allow movement. With time, much like a building exposed to the elements, bones can start to weaken. And for women, this is a real concern, especially as age takes its toll. But here's the silver lining: wall Pilates steps in as a handy tool to help fortify these bones and give them the strength they need.

The Science Behind Bone Health

Before diving into how wall Pilates helps, let's unwrap the basics of bone health. Bones are living tissues, continuously breaking down and rebuilding. This process, called bone remodeling, keeps them healthy and strong. In our early years, bone formation outpaces bone loss, which means bones grow denser. However, as we hit our late twenties, the scales tip the other way. Bone loss starts to outpace formation, leading to a decrease in bone density.

For women, this natural decline becomes more pronounced after menopause. The drop in estrogen levels during this time accelerates bone loss. In some cases, this can lead to osteoporosis, a condition where bones become so fragile that even a minor fall can lead to fractures.

Wall Pilates: The Bone-Strengthening Star

So, where does wall Pilates fit into this picture? Wall Pilates is a weight-bearing exercise, meaning it makes your body work against gravity. This kind of exercise encourages bone-forming cells to spring into action, leading to increased bone density. Think of it as giving your bones a little workout, making them tougher and more resistant to wear and tear.

But that's not all. Wall Pilates, with its focus on posture and alignment, ensures that the weight is distributed evenly across the skeletal system. This reduces the risk of undue pressure on certain bones, thus preventing injuries. It's a holistic approach, taking care of both the bones and the muscles supporting them.

Beyond Just Bones

While the primary focus here is on bones, it's essential to note the added benefits of wall Pilates. This form of exercise, with its controlled movements and emphasis on core strength, promotes better balance. Better balance means a lower risk of falls, which is especially crucial for those with fragile bones. It's a chain reaction; stronger bones and better balance result in increased confidence in daily activities, leading to an active and independent life.

Moreover, wall Pilates doesn't just strengthen the bones of the legs and spine, areas typically targeted by weight-bearing exercises. The varied movements and poses ensure that the entire skeletal system gets a boost. From the arms to the hips, every bone reaps the rewards.

Consistency is Key

With wall Pilates, as with any exercise regimen, it's not a one-and-done deal. Consistency plays a vital role. Making it a regular part of one's routine ensures that the bone-strengthening benefits continue over time. After all, the process of bone remodeling is ongoing. By consistently practicing wall Pilates, one provides a continuous stimulus for bone formation, keeping the threats of age-related bone loss at bay.

A Core of Steel: Goodbye, Mommy Tummy!

The core is the centerpiece of the human body, acting as the central hub from which all our movements originate. It is the powerhouse, the command center, and the origin of our physical strength. And yet, for many women, especially those who have experienced the wonders of motherhood, this central zone can sometimes feel less like a fortress and more like a soft cushion. This softening, often endearingly termed the "mommy tummy," is a natural outcome of childbirth. However, with the right approach, reclaiming a strong and firm core is within reach. Enter wall Pilates, the unsung hero in the quest for a core of steel.

Understanding the Core

Before exploring how wall Pilates can help, it's essential to understand what the core is and why it's so crucial. Contrary to popular belief, the core isn't just the front abdominal muscles. It's a complex network that includes the deep abdominal muscles, back muscles, pelvic floor, and even the diaphragm. This group works in harmony, providing stability, balance, and power for almost every movement we make.

During pregnancy, the core goes through significant changes to accommodate the growing baby. The abdominal muscles stretch, and in some cases, they can even separate—a condition known as diastasis recti. Post-childbirth, many women find that their core feels different. It might seem weaker, less stable, or simply not as firm as before.

Wall Pilates to the Rescue

Wall Pilates offers a solution tailored for strengthening the core, especially post-pregnancy. The exercises in wall Pilates focus on slow, controlled movements, ensuring that the core muscles are engaged throughout. This constant engagement acts as a gentle yet effective workout, targeting the deep muscles that are often overlooked in traditional workouts.

One of the standout features of wall Pilates is its emphasis on the mind-body connection. Every movement is done with intention, with a focus on how it feels. This mindfulness ensures that the core muscles are activated correctly, leading to more effective strengthening over time.

Another advantage of wall Pilates is its adaptability. The exercises can be modified to suit individual needs. For a new mother, this means she can start with gentler exercises and gradually increase intensity as her body heals and strengthens.

Benefits Beyond Strength

While the primary goal might be to say goodbye to the mommy tummy, wall Pilates offers a range of additional benefits. A strong core translates to better posture. This is especially beneficial for mothers who spend a lot of time carrying their babies or bending over during playtime. With a sturdy core, there's less strain on the back, leading to fewer aches and pains.

Additionally, a firm core boosts confidence. It's not just about appearance but also about how one feels. Knowing that the body's central hub is strong gives a sense of empowerment, making daily tasks feel easier and more manageable.

The Road to a Core of Steel

Achieving a core of steel through wall Pilates isn't an overnight process. It requires patience, consistency, and dedication. But the beauty of wall Pilates is that it's a journey of discovery. With every session, one learns more about their body, understanding its strengths and areas that need more attention. Over time, the results become evident, not just in the mirror but in everyday life.

For women who have experienced childbirth, the body goes through a whirlwind of changes. Wall Pilates offers a way to navigate these changes, providing a path to reclaim the body's strength. It's a gentle yet effective approach, ensuring that every woman can find her inner powerhouse, leading to a core that's not just strong but truly made of steel.

The mommy tummy is a badge of honor, a testament to the miracle of life. But with wall Pilates, it's possible to cherish this badge while also working towards a stronger, firmer core. It's the perfect blend of appreciation for what the body has achieved and dedication to making it even stronger for the future.

The Golden Years: Menopause and More

The golden years are often painted in hues of relaxation, wisdom, and the joys of reaping the rewards of years of hard work. But for many women, this phase also brings with it a wave of changes, both physical and emotional. Menopause stands out as one of the most significant milestones during these years. It's a natural part of aging, marking the end of the reproductive years. However, the shift in hormone levels that accompanies menopause can lead to a variety of symptoms, some of which can be quite challenging. Amidst these changes, wall Pilates emerges as a beacon, offering a way to navigate the golden years with grace, strength, and vitality.

Menopause: The Change and Its Effects

Menopause is defined by the cessation of menstrual periods for 12 consecutive months. While it's a natural process, the body's adjustment to decreasing levels of estrogen can lead to several symptoms. These can range from hot flashes, night sweats, and mood swings to more long-term concerns like bone density loss and changes in muscle mass.

Furthermore, the drop in estrogen levels can lead to a reduction in metabolic rate, making it easier for women to gain weight during this period. There's also a shift in where the body stores fat, with a higher tendency to accumulate it around the abdomen.

Wall Pilates: A Friend Through the Changes

Wall Pilates, with its gentle yet effective exercises, offers a solution tailored for the needs of women navigating menopause. Here's how:

- **Bone Health**: As discussed in previous sections, wall Pilates is a weight-bearing exercise, promoting bone density. This is crucial during menopause, where the risk of osteoporosis increases.
- **Muscle Mass**: The exercises in wall Pilates target various muscle groups, helping in maintaining and even building muscle mass. Stronger muscles not only boost metabolism but also provide better support to the joints, reducing the risk of injuries.
- **Mood Elevator**: The focus on controlled breathing and the mind-body connection in wall Pilates can act as a natural mood elevator. The deep breaths stimulate the parasympathetic nervous system, promoting relaxation and reducing stress levels.
- **Flexibility and Balance**: Wall Pilates exercises enhance flexibility, ensuring that the joints remain supple. Additionally, the emphasis on core strength improves balance, crucial in preventing falls.

Navigating the Golden Years with Wall Pilates

Adopting wall Pilates during the golden years is more than just a fitness choice; it's a lifestyle decision. The routines not only address the physical challenges of menopause but also offer a space for relaxation, reflection, and self-care.

The slow, intentional movements allow women to connect with their bodies, understanding and appreciating the changes. It's a celebration of the body's journey, acknowledging the past and preparing for the future.

Furthermore, wall Pilates is adaptable. The exercises can be modified to suit individual needs, ensuring that every woman, regardless of her fitness level, can benefit from them.

A Bright Horizon

The golden years, with all their changes, also bring with them a wealth of experiences, wisdom, and opportunities. With wall Pilates as a trusted companion, women can face the challenges head-on, turning them into opportunities for growth.

In these years, life offers the chance to reflect, to find new passions, and to rediscover old ones. Wall Pilates fits perfectly into this narrative, promoting physical health while also offering a space for mental and emotional well-being.

So, while menopause and the accompanying changes might seem daunting, they don't define the golden years. With tools like wall Pilates, women have the power to shape this phase of their lives, ensuring that it's truly golden in every sense. It's a time of strength, grace, and renewed vitality, promising a horizon that's bright and full of potential.

Chapter 6
Seniors, It's Never Too Late for Wall Pilates!

Growing older brings its own set of challenges. Muscles may not be as spry, balance might teeter a bit more, and flexibility can feel like a thing of the past. But here's the good news: age doesn't have to be a roadblock to feeling strong and vibrant. Enter Wall Pilates, a fantastic way to reignite that youthful energy and revitalize the body.

Wall Pilates isn't just about moving; it's a gift to the body. Think of it as a tool, a friend even, always ready to help bring out the best in physical health. For seniors especially, this method offers a safe and effective means to maintain and improve fitness levels. No need for fancy equipment or gym memberships. Just a sturdy wall, a positive attitude, and a little effort can make a world of difference.

But why Wall Pilates? For one, it helps in enhancing flexibility. With age, the joints might feel a tad stiff. Through gentle stretches and movements against the wall, those joints can regain their former mobility. And that's just the beginning. Balance, often tricky for many seniors, can see marked improvement. No more wobbles or fears of tripping. The exercises focus on strengthening the core, the body's natural stabilizer.

Muscle tone, too, gets a boost. Toned muscles are not just about looks; they play a crucial role in daily activities. Whether it's picking up a grandchild or simply getting out of a chair, strong muscles make everything easier. Lastly, the mind benefits as well. Concentrating on each movement sharpens the mind, providing both mental and physical stimulation.

Let's Get Bendy: Flexibility at Any Age

Flexibility is a gift. Think back to childhood, when bending down to pick up a toy or stretching to reach a high shelf came as naturally as breathing. Over time, though, life happens. Years of sitting, standing, and moving in certain ways can lead to stiff and tight muscles. But here's a nugget of wisdom: age does not have to dictate how flexible one is. With Wall Pilates, rediscovering that ease of movement is entirely possible.

Wall Pilates focuses on gentle movements and stretches. These exercises, when done regularly, can work wonders on the muscles and joints. They help release tension, making the body feel more open and freer. And the best part? No need for fancy props or complicated routines. A plain wall is the perfect partner.

The Science Behind Flexibility

At a basic level, flexibility refers to the range of motion in the joints and the ability of the muscles to stretch. Two main components play a role in this: the muscles themselves and the tendons (the stretchy bands connecting muscles to bones). Over time, without regular stretching, these can become tight and short. This tightness can make everyday tasks more challenging and can even lead to discomfort or pain.

Wall Pilates exercises focus on lengthening these muscles and tendons. By doing so, they help increase the range of motion in the joints. This means easier movement and a greater sense of freedom in the body.

Benefits of Being Flexible

Increased flexibility offers a plethora of benefits. For starters, daily tasks become simpler. Bending to tie a shoe, reaching for something on a high shelf, or turning to look over one's shoulder while driving – all these activities become easier. Beyond that, flexibility can reduce the risk of injuries. When the muscles are supple, they are less prone to strains and sprains.

A flexible body also means better posture. Tight muscles can pull the body out of its natural alignment, leading to slouched or hunched shoulders. By stretching and strengthening the right muscles, Wall Pilates can help correct these imbalances, leading to a more upright and confident stance.

Wall Pilates and Flexibility

So, how does Wall Pilates help improve flexibility? These exercises use the support of a wall to guide and deepen stretches. For instance, a simple calf stretch becomes more effective when done against a wall. The firm surface provides feedback, allowing one to adjust and get the most out of each stretch.

Another advantage is that the wall provides stability. This means that even those who might be worried about balance can stretch with confidence. They can focus entirely on the stretch without the fear of toppling over.

Tips for Maximum Flexibility Gains

1. **Consistency is Key**: Like any other form of exercise, the benefits of Wall Pilates come with regular practice. It's not about how long each session is but rather how often it's done. Even a few minutes every day can lead to noticeable improvements.
2. **Listen to the Body**: This cannot be stressed enough. Everybody is different. While stretching, it's essential to pay attention to how it feels. A gentle pull is good, but pain is a signal to ease off.
3. **Breathe**: It might sound simple but breathing plays a crucial role in flexibility. Deep, even breaths can help relax the muscles, making them more receptive to stretching.
4. **Stay Hydrated**: Muscles work best when they are well-hydrated. Drinking enough water ensures that they remain supple and elastic.
5. **Warm-Up**: Jumping straight into deep stretches is not the best idea. A short warm-up, like a brisk walk or some gentle movements, prepares the muscles and makes them more pliable.

Age is just a number, especially when it comes to flexibility. With the right tools and approach, like Wall Pilates, anyone can enjoy the benefits of a supple and mobile body. It's about taking small steps every day, listening to one's body, and enjoying the process. After all, flexibility is not just about the body's ability to bend and stretch; it's also about adapting, growing, and making the most of every moment. And with Wall Pilates, that's entirely within reach.

Wobble No More: Balance and Coordination

Balance is a subtle art. As kids, most people could hop on one foot or spin around without a second thought. As the years go by, however, the sure-footedness of youth might give way to moments of unsteadiness. A missed step here, a small stumble there, and suddenly balance becomes something on the mind. But the good news is, with Wall Pilates, that stability can be reclaimed.

Understanding Balance and Coordination

At its core, balance is the ability to maintain the body's center of mass over its base of support. Several systems in the body work together to make this happen. The visual system (eyes), the vestibular system (ears), and the proprioceptive system (sensors in the muscles and joints) all send information to the brain, which then directs the muscles on how to move.

Coordination, on the other hand, is the ability to move different parts of the body smoothly and efficiently. It's what allows a person to walk without thinking, to climb stairs, or to catch a falling object.

The Role of Wall Pilates

Wall Pilates, with its emphasis on core strength and controlled movements, is a powerful tool for enhancing both balance and coordination. The wall acts as a steady partner, offering support and feedback. It's there to lean on, to push against, and to provide that extra bit of confidence.

The exercises in Wall Pilates focus on strengthening the muscles that stabilize the body, especially those in the core. A strong core is like a sturdy anchor, keeping the body upright and steady. The movements also train the muscles to work together in harmony, which is the essence of coordination.

1. **Safety**: One of the most immediate benefits is a reduced risk of falls. Better balance means fewer stumbles and trips. This is especially important for seniors, as falls can lead to serious injuries.
2. **Efficiency in Daily Tasks**: From walking to reaching for objects, improved coordination makes every movement more fluid and effortless.
3. **Enhanced Athletic Performance**: For those who enjoy sports or other physical activities, good balance and coordination can boost performance and enjoyment.
4. **Increased Body Awareness**: Wall Pilates exercises require attention to how the body moves. Over time, this leads to a heightened sense of body awareness, making it easier to adjust and correct posture and movement.

Tips for Better Balance and Coordination

1. **Practice Regularly**: Just like any other skill, balance and coordination improve with practice. Regular Wall Pilates sessions can lead to steady improvements.
2. **Focus on the Core**: The core muscles, which include the abdominals, back, and pelvis, play a central role in maintaining balance. Exercises that strengthen these muscles can have a big impact.
3. **Challenge the Body**: Over time, as balance improves, it's beneficial to introduce new challenges. This could be as simple as closing the eyes during a balance exercise or trying a slightly more advanced movement.
4. **Stay Active**: Outside of Wall Pilates, staying active in general can help. Activities like walking, dancing, or even standing on one foot while brushing teeth can all contribute to better balance.
5. **Mind the Feet**: The feet are the body's foundation. Taking care of them, wearing supportive shoes, and even doing foot-strengthening exercises can make a difference.

Balance and coordination are skills that can be honed and refined at any age. With the help of Wall Pilates, everyone has the opportunity to move with more grace, stability, and confidence. It's a chance to rediscover the joy of movement, to feel more connected to the body, and to embrace each day with a steady stride. So, with the support of a trusty wall and a bit of effort, wobbles and stumbles can become a thing of the past.

Muscle Matters: Keep That Tone

Muscles are quite the marvels. They lift, pull, push, and carry, making every movement possible. From the powerful muscles that help stand and walk, to the smaller ones that allow for intricate hand gestures, each plays a critical role in daily life. As time passes, however, these muscles may lose some of their vigor and vitality. But here comes the silver lining: Wall Pilates offers a way to rekindle that muscle strength and tone.

The Basics of Muscle Tone

Muscle tone isn't just about how muscles look, but how they function. It refers to the tension in a muscle when it's at rest. Good muscle tone means muscles are responsive and ready to spring into action. They support the body, maintain posture, and provide strength for movements, both big and small.

As age advances, muscle mass naturally decreases, and without regular exercise, what remains can become weaker and less toned. This can affect not just strength, but also balance, coordination, and metabolism.

Why Wall Pilates Makes a Difference

Wall Pilates stands out as a method to help maintain and even improve muscle tone. Here's how:

1. **Targeted Exercises:** Wall Pilates exercises are designed to target specific muscle groups. Whether it's the muscles of the core, the legs, or the arms, each exercise focuses on strengthening and toning effectively.
2. **Resistance:** The wall, although a simple structure, provides a form of resistance. Pushing or pulling against it engages the muscles, making them work harder.

3. **Controlled Movements:** Wall Pilates emphasizes controlled, deliberate movements. This control engages the muscles for longer, boosting both strength and endurance.

4. **Versatility:** With a variety of exercises to choose from, Wall Pilates offers options for every fitness level. This means that as strength and tone improve, the exercises can be adapted to offer more challenge.

Benefits of Maintaining Muscle Tone

5. **Daily Life Becomes Easier:** Strong, toned muscles make everyday activities smoother. Whether it's carrying groceries, climbing stairs, or playing with grandchildren, good muscle tone provides the strength needed.

6. **Improved Metabolism:** Muscles, even at rest, burn more calories than fat. So, the more muscle tone one has, the higher the resting metabolic rate. This can be beneficial for weight management.

7. **Better Bone Health:** Regular strength exercises, like Wall Pilates, can help increase bone density. This is especially important for post-menopausal women, who are at a higher risk of osteoporosis.

8. **Enhanced Posture:** Strong muscles support the spine and hold the body upright. This means fewer aches and pains and a more confident appearance.

Tips to Maximize Muscle Tone with Wall Pilates

1. **Consistency:** Regular practice is essential. Even short sessions, done consistently, can lead to improvements in muscle tone.

2. **Full Range of Motion:** When doing each exercise, moving through the full range of motion ensures that the muscles are worked thoroughly.

3. **Stay Hydrated:** Water supports muscle function. Drinking enough ensures that muscles work optimally.

4. **Rest and Recovery**: Muscles grow and repair during rest. So, it's essential to give them time to recover after a Wall Pilates session.

5. **Mix It Up:** Variety is not just the spice of life; it's also essential for muscles. Changing up the exercises every so often can prevent plateaus and keep the muscles engaged.

With Wall Pilates, the opportunity to keep them strong and toned is within grasp. It's a gentle nudge, a reminder that no matter the age, the body is capable of strength and vitality. So, with the help of a trusty wall and some dedication, muscles can remain robust and ready for all of life's adventures.

Brain Gains: Because Pilates Isn't Just Physical

Pilates, especially the Wall Pilates variety, offers more than just a path to physical fitness. While the muscles, joints, and bones undoubtedly benefit, there's another crucial part of the body that reaps rewards: the brain. The connection between physical activity and brain health is compelling, and Wall Pilates sits at the intersection of this exciting relationship.

The Brain-Body Link

The brain and body are deeply interconnected. Every movement made, whether it's a simple blink or a complex dance step, starts as a thought. The brain sends signals through the nervous system, directing the muscles on what to do. Conversely, as the body moves and senses its environment, it sends a flood of information back to the brain.

Wall Pilates, with its focus on controlled movements and body awareness, strengthens this two-way communication. Each exercise requires concentration and attention to detail, forging new neural pathways and reinforcing existing ones.

Benefits for the Brain

Engaging in Wall Pilates offers a treasure trove of benefits for the brain:

1. **Enhanced Cognitive Function**: Regular physical activity, including Pilates, has been shown to boost cognitive functions like memory, attention, and problem-solving. The brain becomes more agile, better equipped to handle challenges.
2. **Stress Reduction**: Stress is a part of life, but chronic stress can be harmful to the brain. The mindful nature of Wall Pilates, combined with the physical exertion, can help reduce stress levels. As the body moves and stretches, tension melts away, and the mind becomes calmer.

3. **Improved Mood**: Physical activity releases endorphins, the body's feel-good chemicals. These can help reduce feelings of sadness or anxiety, leading to a brighter mood and a more positive outlook on life.
4. **Better Sleep**: Quality sleep is crucial for brain health. It's the time when the brain processes information, forms memories, and heals. Regular Wall Pilates sessions can lead to better sleep quality and duration.
5. **Increased Brain Plasticity**: Plasticity refers to the brain's ability to change and adapt. Every time a new movement is learned in Wall Pilates, the brain forms new connections. This adaptability is essential for learning and memory.

Principles of Wall Pilates and Brain Health

Wall Pilates is grounded in several principles, many of which directly support brain health:

1. **Concentration**: Each exercise demands focus. This act of concentrating not only enhances the effectiveness of the movement but also gives the brain a workout.
2. **Control**: Wall Pilates is not about fast or forceful movements. It's about control. This control requires coordination between the brain and muscles, strengthening their connection.
3. **Precision**: Precision in movement means attention to detail. It's this precision that ensures the exercises are effective and safe. For the brain, it means a constant stream of feedback, refining and adjusting movements as needed.
4. **Breathing**: Deep, rhythmic breathing is a cornerstone of Wall Pilates. Breathing brings oxygen to the brain, supporting its function. It also promotes relaxation and stress reduction.
5. **Flow**: The exercises in Wall Pilates flow smoothly from one to the next. This flow requires planning and foresight, skills that engage and challenge the brain.

Wall Pilates is a celebration of the brain-body connection. It's an invitation to move, to think, and to feel in harmony. While the physical benefits, like improved muscle tone and flexibility, are evident, the brain gains are equally significant. With every stretch, push, and pull, the brain becomes a bit sharper, a bit more resilient, and a lot more vibrant.

Chapter 7
Creating Your Very Own Wall Pilates Space

Imagine a space, a special corner in your home, dedicated solely to your well-being. A place where the body stretches, strengthens, and finds harmony. This dream can be a reality, and the beauty of Wall Pilates is that it doesn't demand much. No sprawling rooms or expensive equipment. Just a little bit of space, a sturdy wall, and a commitment to oneself.

The beauty of Wall Pilates lies in its simplicity and accessibility. Whether living in a spacious home or a cozy apartment, creating a dedicated Pilates space is achievable for everyone. This chapter will guide you through the essentials of setting up that perfect spot. From selecting the right wall to ensuring safety, every step is designed to make the Wall Pilates experience smooth and enjoyable.

The journey towards health and wellness is unique for each person. Yet, having a special place in the home that resonates with calm and positivity can make a world of difference. This space becomes a sanctuary, a reminder to pause, breathe, and care for oneself. So, as we explore the ins and outs of crafting this Pilates haven, remember that it's more than just a physical setup. It's a commitment to self-care, a promise of many fulfilling sessions of stretching, strengthening, and rejuvenating the mind and body.

What You Will Need (Spoiler: Not Much!)

Wall Pilates, in its essence, is about embracing simplicity and making the most of what's available. The magic of this exercise form lies in its minimalism. No need for a dedicated room filled with expensive gear. A few basic items and a touch of commitment are all that's required. Let's explore the modest list of essentials to kickstart the Wall Pilates journey.

1. *The Right Wall*

Arguably the most crucial component for Wall Pilates is, well, a wall. But not just any wall will do. What's needed is a clear, sturdy space free from obstructions like furniture, decorations, or windows. The ideal wall:

- Should be flat and smooth. Avoid walls with significant textures or protruding designs.
- Must be strong enough to withstand pressure from exercises. Most interior walls will suffice, but always ensure the wall's integrity.
- A minimum width of about four feet and a height that matches the user's full reach when their arms are extended overhead.

2. *Supportive Footwear*

While many Pilates exercises are done barefoot, for Wall Pilates, consider using supportive footwear. This can provide better grip and support during exercises. Opt for:

- Shoes with non-slip soles.
- Comfortable fit, neither too tight nor too loose.
- Lightweight shoes that don't restrict movement.

3. *Comfortable Attire*

Wear clothing that allows freedom of movement. It's essential to feel comfortable and unrestricted during exercises. Some recommendations include:

- Stretchable pants or leggings.
- Breathable tops that aren't too baggy. You wouldn't want your clothing to get in the way of your movements or obscure your form.
- Avoid belts, large jewelry, or anything that might interfere with exercises or scratch the wall.

4. *A Soft Mat*

For exercises that require sitting or lying down, a soft mat can provide comfort. It can also offer grip and define your workout space. When choosing a mat:

- Opt for one that's thick enough to cushion and protect your spine, but not so thick that it's unstable.
- Ensure it's made of a non-slip material for safety.

- It should be easy to clean and store away.

5. A Small Towel

A towel can serve multiple purposes:

- It can provide a cushion between you and the wall for certain exercises.
- Useful for wiping away sweat.
- Can serve as a grip aid for some stretches.

6. Resistance Bands (Optional)

While not a strict requirement, resistance bands can add variety and intensity to some exercises. They're lightweight, affordable, and versatile. If considering resistance bands:

- Have a few with different resistance levels.
- Ensure they're free from tears or wear that might cause them to snap.

7. A Mirror (Optional)

Installing a mirror opposite your workout space can be beneficial. It allows for:

- Checking form and posture during exercises.
- Providing visual feedback to adjust and correct movements in real-time.

8. Hydration

Always have a bottle of water nearby. Staying hydrated supports muscle function and aids recovery.

9. A Notebook or Journal

While not a piece of physical exercise equipment, having a place to jot down routines, track progress, and note any challenges or achievements can be incredibly motivating.

The beauty of Wall Pilates shines through its simplicity. The few items on this list are easy to find and, in many cases, already present in most homes. Setting up the perfect Wall Pilates space is less about accumulating things and more about creating a dedicated spot where focus, effort, and transformation converge. With these basics in place, the stage is set for a fulfilling and rejuvenating Wall Pilates experience.

Safety First, Always

Safety is the cornerstone of any fitness practice. In the realm of Wall Pilates, while the exercises are designed to be gentle and accessible, it's paramount to ensure that every move is made safely. After all, the goal is to enhance well-being, not jeopardize it. This chapter will shed light on the vital safety measures and best practices to keep in mind while indulging in Wall Pilates.

Understanding the Importance of Safety

Every exercise regimen carries with it inherent risks. A misstep, an overstretch, or even a momentary lapse in focus can lead to injuries. Wall Pilates, with its reliance on the wall for support, minimizes many risks, but it's still essential to approach each session with caution. Ensuring safety means ensuring continuity in practice and reaping the long-term benefits of Wall Pilates.

Key Safety Measures for Wall Pilates

1. **Know the Body's Limits**: It's essential to understand personal physical limitations. If any movement feels painful or overly strenuous, it's a signal to stop. Pain is the body's way of indicating something isn't right.
2. **Warm Up Properly**: Jumping straight into exercises without a proper warm-up can strain cold muscles. Dedicate the first few minutes of each session to gentle stretches and breathing exercises to get the blood flowing and prepare the body.
3. **Ensure the Wall is Sturdy**: Before starting, give the chosen wall a good inspection. It should be free from any damage, cracks, or dampness. Push against it with some force to ensure it can withstand the pressure.
4. **Keep the Area Clear**: The immediate area around the wall should be free from any obstructions like furniture or loose items. This ensures there's enough space to move freely and reduces the risk of tripping or getting hurt.
5. **Maintain a Steady Base**: For exercises that require standing, ensure the feet are firmly planted on the ground. If using a mat, it should be non-slip. Stable footing is the foundation of safe Wall Pilates exercises.

6. **Stay Hydrated**: Muscles work best when they're hydrated. Drink water before, during, and after the session to keep muscles supple and responsive.

7. **Focus on Form**: Proper form is crucial. It ensures that the right muscles are targeted and reduces the risk of strain or injury. If unsure about the correct form, it might be helpful to consult a Pilates instructor or reliable resources.

8. **Use Props Wisely**: If using props like resistance bands, always check them for wear and tear before use. A snapped band can cause injuries.

9. **Listen to Feedback**: The body is constantly giving feedback. A stretch that feels good, a muscle working hard, or a twinge of pain – it's all valuable information. Always pay attention to these signals and adjust movements accordingly.

10. **Cool Down**: Just as warming up is essential, so is cooling down. Dedicate the last few minutes of each session to slowing the heart rate and relaxing the muscles. Gentle stretches and deep breathing can aid this process.

Special Considerations for Seniors

1. For seniors or those with specific health conditions, there are a few additional precautions:

2. **Consult a Doctor**: Before starting Wall Pilates or any exercise regimen, it's wise to consult with a healthcare professional, especially if there are existing health concerns.

3. **Avoid Overexertion**: It's okay to take things slow. The aim should be steady progress, not instant results.

4. **Stay Mindful of Chronic Conditions**: Conditions like arthritis or osteoporosis require special attention. Some exercises might need adjustments to ensure they're safe and comfortable.

5. So, while Wall Pilates offers a world of benefits, it's essential to approach it with safety at the forefront. A cautious approach not only prevents injuries but also ensures that the practice is sustainable and enjoyable in the long run. With the right precautions in place, Wall Pilates becomes a safe haven of health, strength, and well-being.

Finding Your Perfect Wall

At the heart of Wall Pilates is, unsurprisingly, a wall. But not all walls are created equal. The wall chosen for Wall Pilates exercises will play a significant role in the effectiveness and safety of the routines. This chapter will guide you through the process of selecting the best wall in your living space, ensuring it meets the criteria for a safe and effective workout.

The Ideal Wall: Key Features

When thinking about Wall Pilates, the wall becomes more than just a structural component of a house. It transforms into a support system, a workout partner, and a canvas for growth. Here are the essential features of the perfect wall:

1. **Sturdy and Solid**: The wall must withstand the pressures and forces exerted during exercises. It should be free from any structural damages, cracks, or signs of wear and tear. While most interior walls in homes are designed to bear weight, it's a good practice to test the wall's sturdiness by gently pushing against it.
2. **Smooth Surface**: A smooth surface ensures that there's no friction or discomfort during exercises. Walls with excessive textures, protruding designs, or irregularities might hinder movements and cause discomfort.
3. **Clear and Unobstructed**: The chosen wall should be free from any obstructions. This includes shelves, artwork, windows, or heating elements. A clear space ensures unrestricted movement and reduces the risk of accidents.
4. **Good Height and Width**: The wall should be tall enough to accommodate full body stretches. In terms of width, a space of at least four feet is ideal to perform a range of exercises without feeling confined.
5. **Easily Cleanable**: With regular workouts, it's likely the wall will need occasional cleaning from sweat or contact. Choosing a wall with a surface that's easy to wipe down can make maintenance hassle-free.

Factors to Consider

While the above features outline the ideal specifications, other factors might influence the choice of wall:

1. **Room Layout**: Consider the layout of the room. Is there enough space around the wall to move freely? Remember, while the wall is the primary support, the surrounding area is equally crucial for exercises that require more space.
2. **Flooring**: The type of flooring in front of the wall can influence comfort and safety. A soft, non-slip floor is ideal. If the floor is too hard, like tile, using a mat can provide cushioning. If it's carpeted, ensure it's taut and not a tripping hazard.
3. **Lighting**: Proper lighting can make exercises easier and safer. A well-lit space ensures that you can see clearly, reducing the risk of missteps or poor form.
4. **Ventilation**: If the room gets too stuffy or hot, it can become uncomfortable to exercise. Ensure the room has good ventilation, either through windows, fans, or air conditioning.
5. **Ambiance**: While not a strict requirement, the ambiance can play a role in motivation and enjoyment. A calm, pleasant environment can make workouts more enjoyable. Consider the wall's color, the view (if there's a window nearby), and any potential distractions.

Temporary Adjustments

If the perfect wall is elusive, temporary adjustments can help:

1. **Wall Protectors**: If concerned about marks or sweat on the wall, using removable wall protectors or washable decals can be a solution.
2. **Portable Barres**: For exercises that require a barre, portable and adjustable barres are available. They can be fixed to the wall during workouts and removed afterward.
3. **Temporary Lighting**: If the room's lighting isn't sufficient, using portable lamps or clip-on lights can help.

The quest for the perfect wall for Wall Pilates is a blend of practicality and personal preference. While structural integrity and safety are paramount, personal comfort and ambiance play a role in creating an inviting workout space. With a bit of observation and possibly some minor adjustments, any home can boast the perfect wall, setting the stage for many enriching Wall Pilates sessions.

Chapter 8
First Steps: The ABCs of Wall Pilates

Stepping into the world of Wall Pilates is like opening a door to newfound strength, flexibility, and balance. These exercises, though simple, pack a punch in terms of benefits. This chapter unveils the basic moves that form the foundation of Wall Pilates. Designed for beginners, yet versatile enough for seasoned practitioners, these exercises introduce the body to the unique dynamics of using a wall for Pilates.

The beauty of these exercises lies in their adaptability. They can be tweaked to be more challenging or toned down based on individual needs. So, without further ado, let's dive into the first set of Wall Pilates exercises.

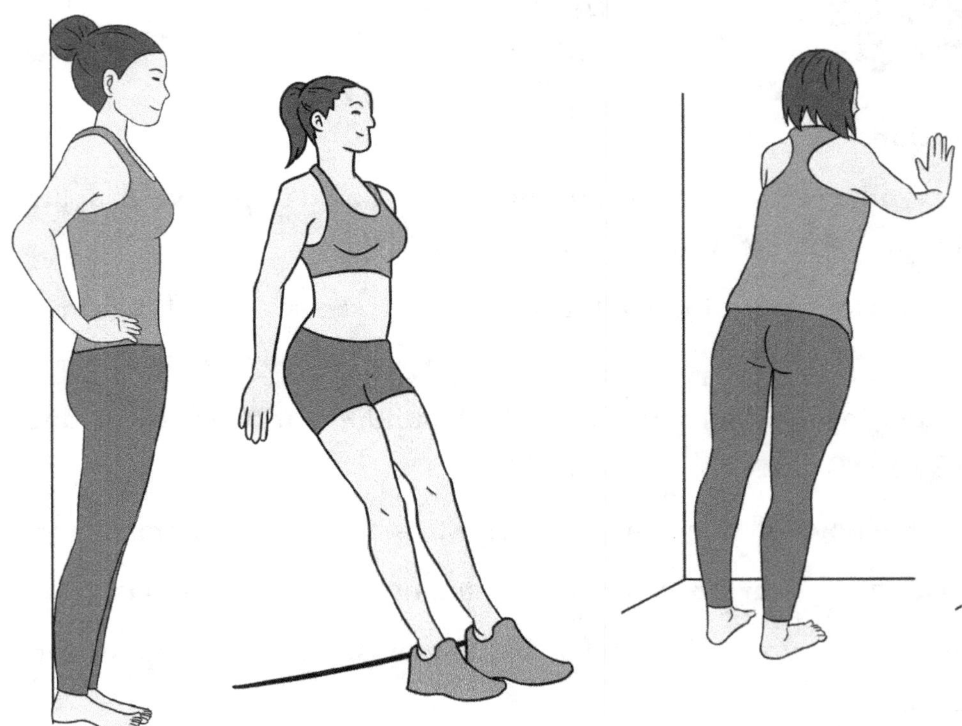

Your First Wall Squat

Objective: Strengthen the thighs and glutes while enhancing lower body stability.

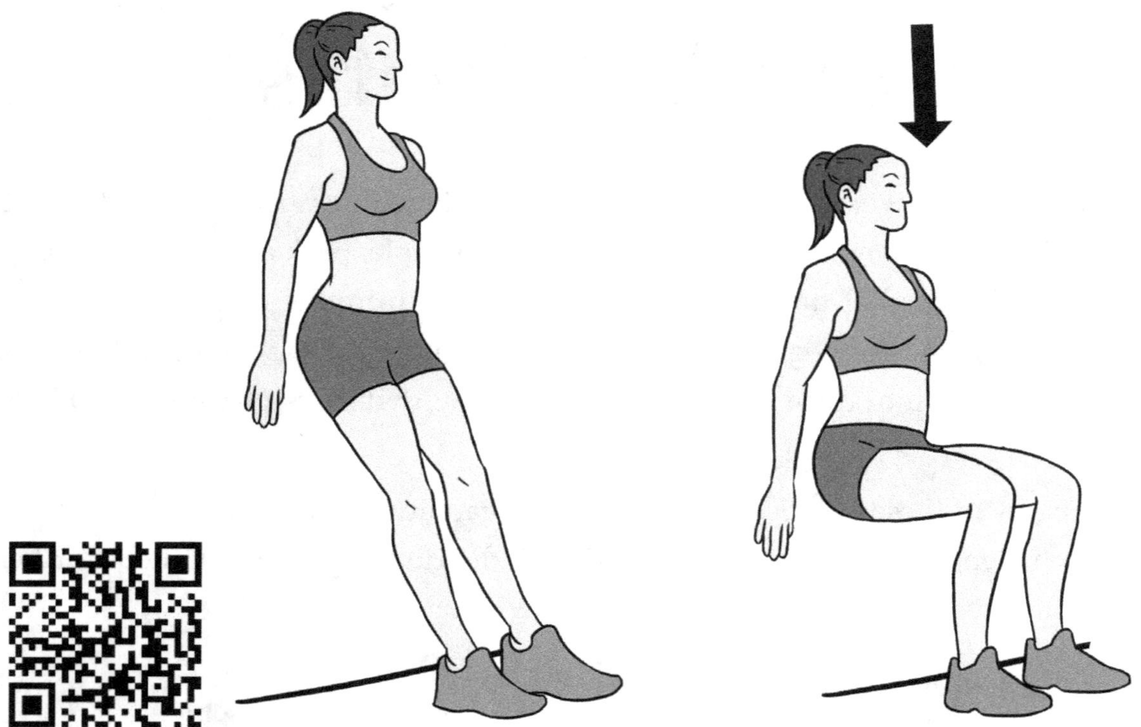

Instructions:

a. Stand with your back against the wall. Feet should be hip-width apart and about a foot away from the wall.

b. Slowly slide down the wall, bending your knees as if sitting on an invisible chair.

c. Aim to bring the thighs parallel to the ground, ensuring knees are directly above the ankles.

d. Hold the position briefly, then slowly slide back up to the starting position.

e. Repeat the motion for the recommended number of repetitions.

Safety Tips: Ensure the back remains flat against the wall. Keep the core engaged.

Repetitions: 10 reps, 2 sets

Push-Ups Without Breaking a Sweat

Objective: Strengthen the arms, chest, and shoulders.

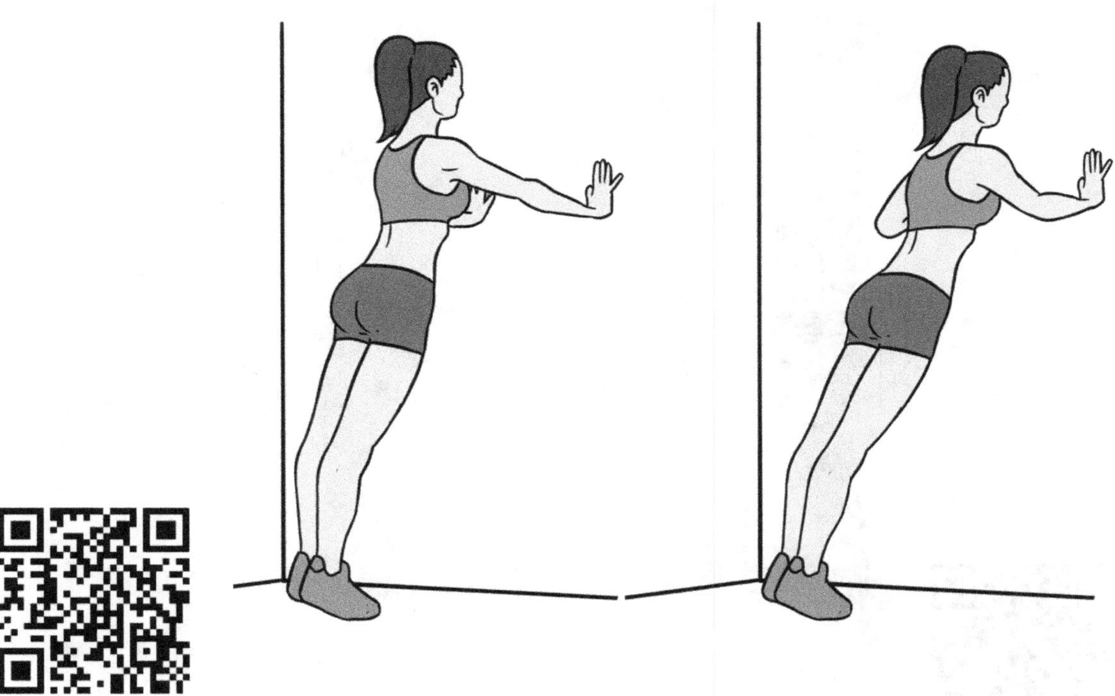

Instructions:

a. Stand facing the wall at arm's length distance.

b. Place palms flat against the wall at shoulder height.

c. Inhale as you bend your elbows and bring your chest closer to the wall.

d. Exhale as you push back to the starting position.

e. Repeat the motion for the recommended number of repetitions.

Safety Tips: Keep the body in a straight line from head to heels.

Repetitions: 10-12 reps, 2 sets

Standing Leg Lifts

Objective: Strengthen and tone the outer thighs and hips.

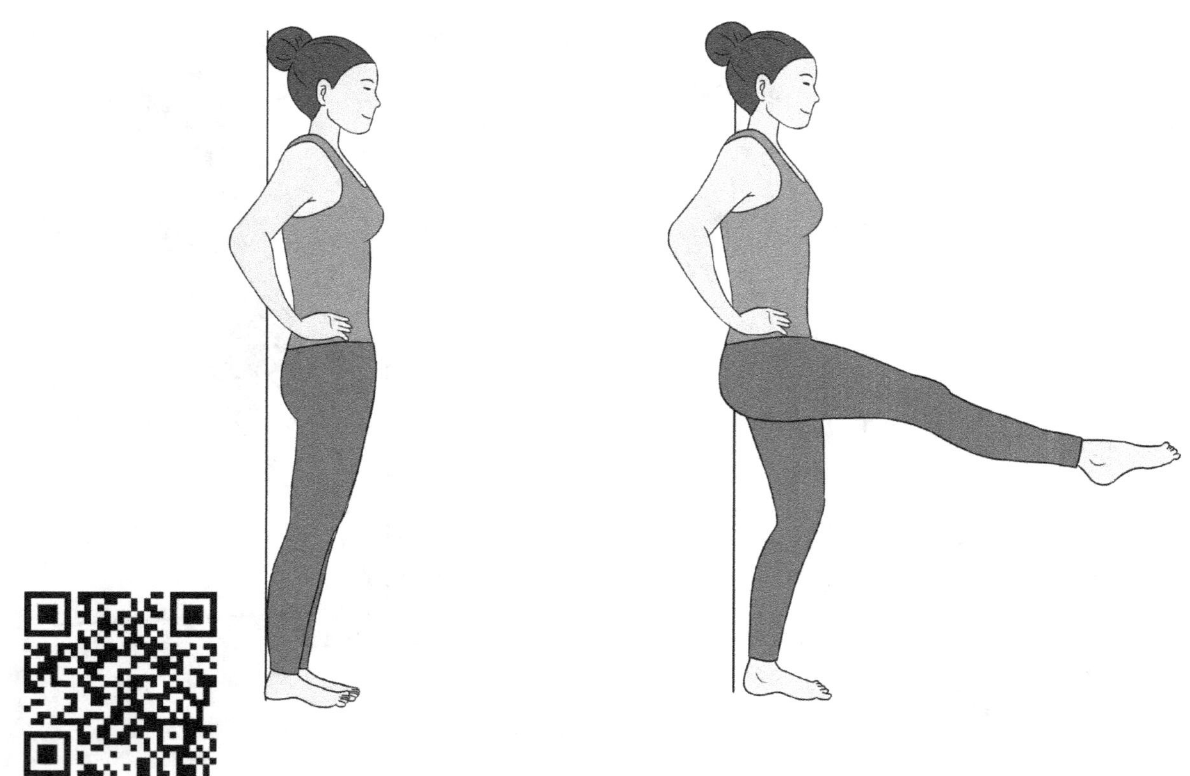

Instructions:

a. Stand sideways to the wall, about an arm's length away.

b. Place your hand on the wall for support.

c. Keeping the leg straight, lift it out to the side as high as comfortably possible.

d. Lower it back down with control.

e. Repeat on the other side after the set is complete.

Safety Tips: Keep the core engaged and avoid leaning too much into the wall.

Repetitions: 10 reps on each side, 2 sets

Wall-assisted Pelvic Tilts

Objective: Strengthen the core and improve lower back flexibility.

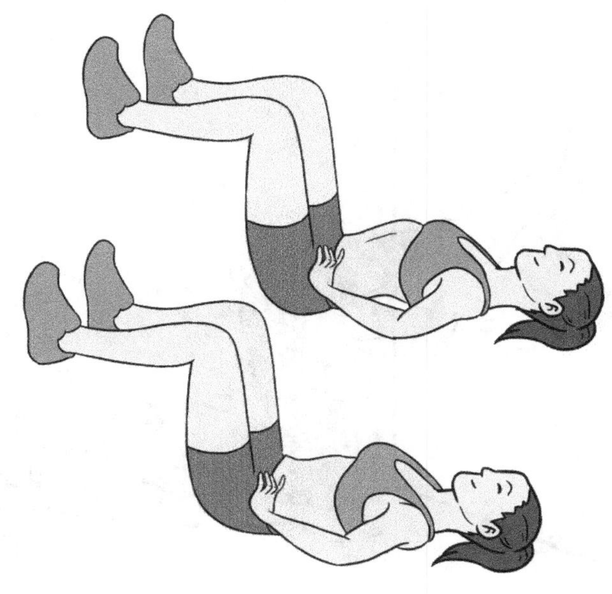

Instructions:

a. Lie on the floor with your back flat, buttocks close to the wall, and legs extended up against it.

Keep feet hip-width apart, pressing gently against the wall.

Engage your core and tilt your pelvis upwards, flattening your lower back against the floor.

Hold the tilt and core engagement for a few seconds, slightly lifting your hips.

Gently relax the tilt, returning your pelvis to its starting position with a natural spine curve.

Perform 2-3 sets of 10-15 repetitions each.

Safety Tips: Move slowly and avoid straining the back.

Repetitions: 10 reps, 2 sets

Wall-assisted Toe Taps

Objective: Strengthen the lower abdominals and improve hip mobility.

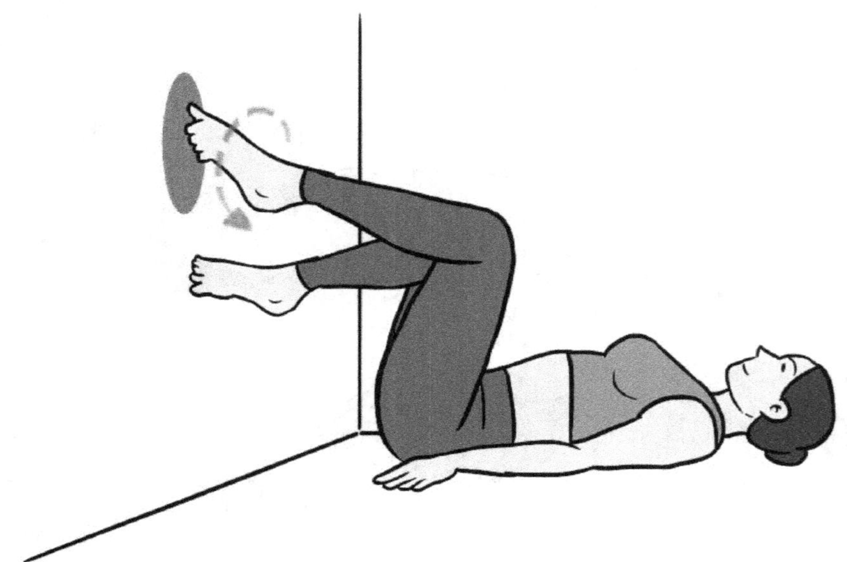

Instructions:

a. Lie on the floor with your legs up and feet flat against the wall. Knees should be bent at a 90-degree angle.

b. Engage the core and slowly lower one foot towards the ground, tapping the toes.

c. Lift the foot back up to the starting position.

d. Repeat with the other foot.

e. Continue alternating feet for the recommended number of repetitions.

Safety Tips: Ensure the lower back remains pressed to the floor.

Repetitions: 10 taps on each foot, 2 sets

Wall-assisted Chest Opener Stretch

Objective: Improve upper body flexibility, especially across the chest and shoulders.

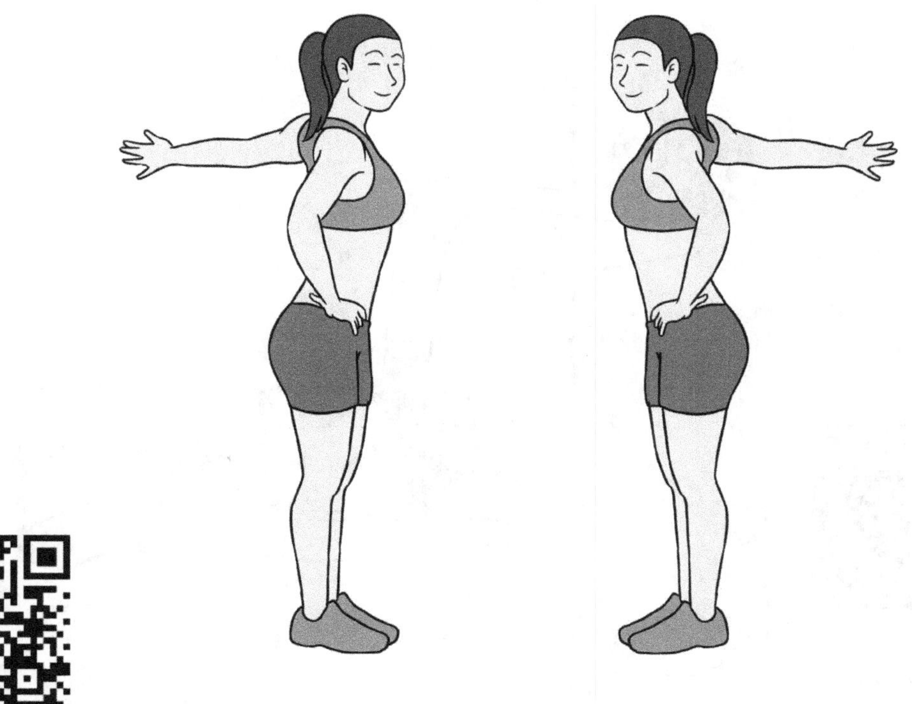

Instructions:

a. Stand sideways near the wall.

b. Extend the arm closest to the wall out and place the palm and forearm flat against it.

c. Slowly turn the body away from the wall until a stretch is felt across the chest.

d. Hold this position for a few breaths, feeling the stretch deepen.

e. Switch sides and repeat.

Safety Tips: Ensure the arm is at shoulder height. Do not overstretch; the movement should be comfortable.

Repetitions: Hold for 20-30 seconds on each side, 2 rounds.

Wall Bridge Preps

Objective: Strengthen the glutes, hamstrings, and lower back.

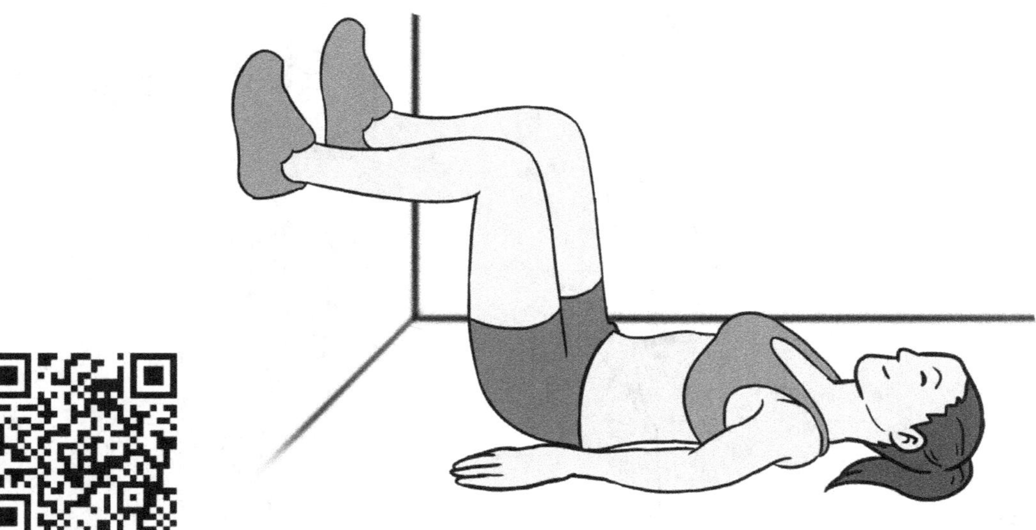

Instructions:

a. Lie on the floor with knees bent and feet flat against the wall.

b. Arms should rest by the sides.

c. Push through the feet and lift the hips off the ground, pressing the lower back into the floor.

d. Hold at the top for a moment, squeezing the glutes.

e. Slowly lower the hips back down. f. Repeat for the recommended number of repetitions.

Safety Tips: Ensure the feet are hip width apart on the wall. Engage the core throughout the movement.

Repetitions: 12-15 reps, 2 sets.

Wall-assisted Knee Raises

Objective: Strengthen the lower abdominals and hip flexors.

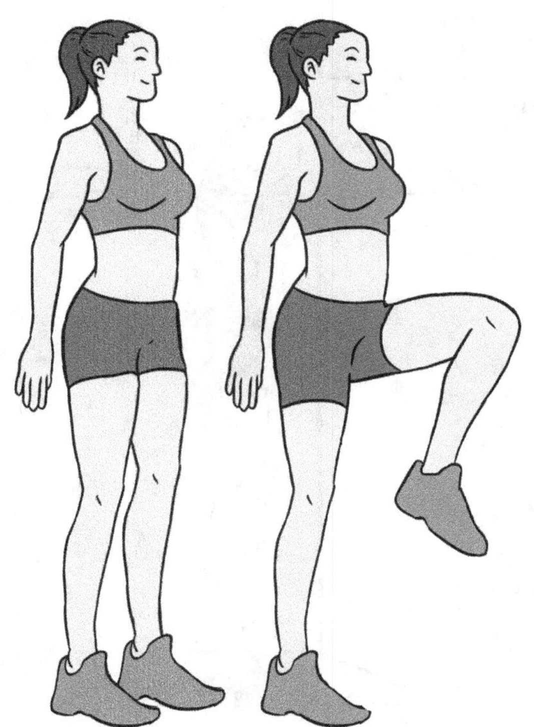

Instructions:

a. Stand facing the wall, about an arm's length away.

b. Place both palms flat on the wall for support.

c. Keeping the core engaged, lift one knee up towards the chest.

d. Lower it back down with control.

e. Repeat with the other leg. f. Continue alternating for the recommended number of repetitions.

Safety Tips: Keep the back straight and avoid leaning too much into the wall.

Repetitions: 10 raises on each leg, 2 sets.

Standing Wall-assisted Cat-Cow Stretch

Objective: Improve flexibility and mobility of the spine.

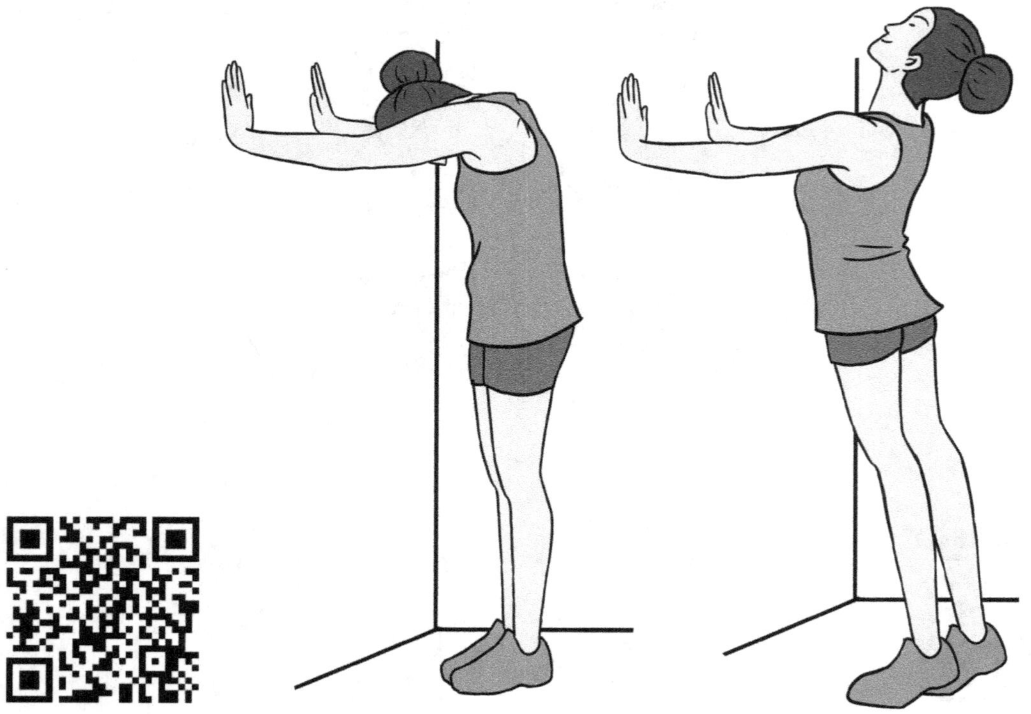

Instructions:

a. Stand facing the wall, about an arm's length away.

b. Place both palms flat on the wall, arms extended.

c. Inhale as you arch the back, lifting the head and tailbone towards the ceiling (Cow position).

d. Exhale as you round the spine, tucking the chin and tailbone (Cat position).

e. Continue moving between these two positions for the recommended number of repetitions.

Safety Tips: Ensure movements are slow and controlled. Focus on moving the spine.

Repetitions: 10 rounds (cat and cow combined), 2 sets.

Wall-assisted Supine Leg Slides

Objective: Strengthen the core, especially the lower abdominals.

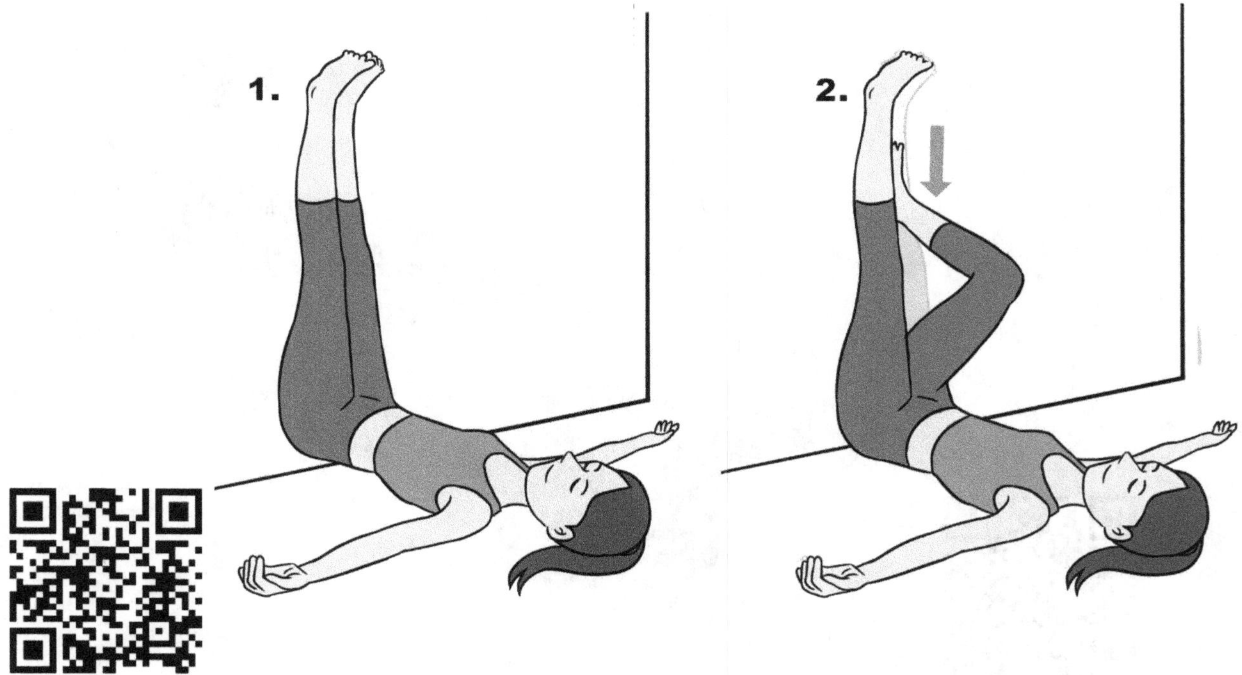

Instructions:

a. Lie on the back with legs extended upwards and feet flat against the wall.

b. Keeping one leg still, slowly slide the other leg down the wall until it's straight and parallel to the floor.

c. Slide the leg back up the wall to meet the other foot.

d. Repeat with the other leg.

e. Continue alternating for the recommended number of repetitions.

Safety Tips: Engage the core throughout the exercise. Ensure the lower back remains pressed to the floor.

Repetitions: 10 slides on each leg, 2 sets.

Wall-assisted Dead Bug

Objective: To activate the core muscles and improve coordination.

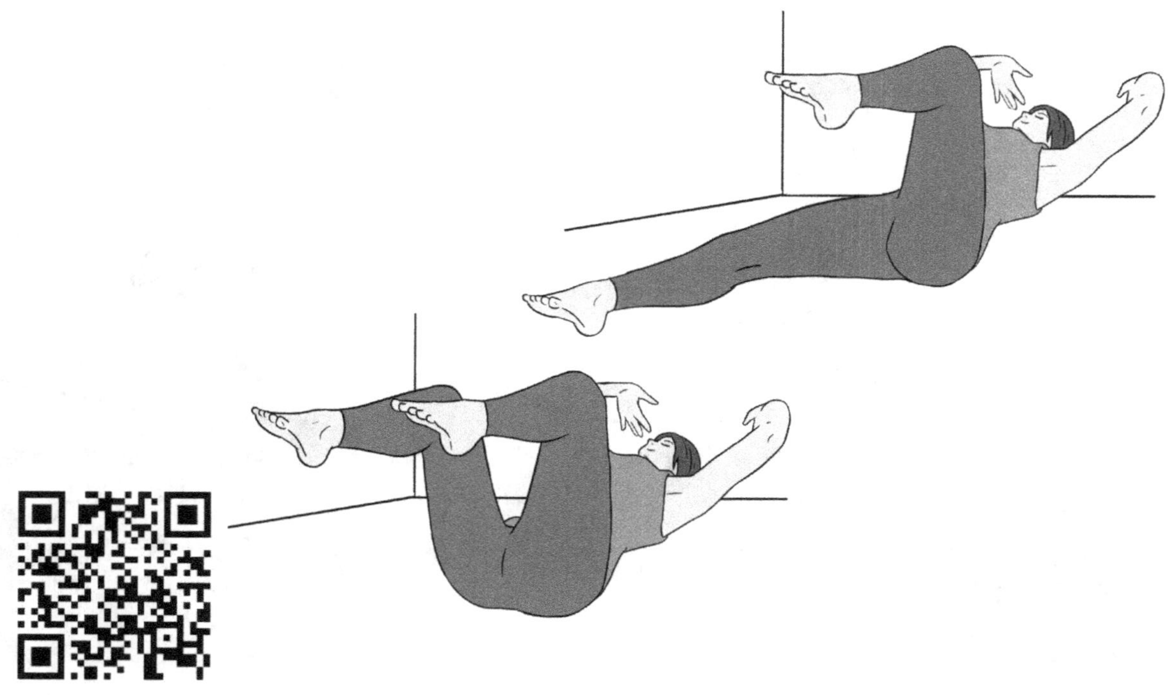

Instructions:

a. Lie flat on your back on the floor, facing up.

b. Raise your arms straight up towards the ceiling.

c. Bend your knees to a 90-degree angle, calves parallel to the floor.

d. Slowly extend your right arm back behind your head while simultaneously straightening your left leg out in front of you.

e. Return to the starting position and repeat with the opposite arm and leg. f. Continue alternating sides for the recommended number of repetitions.

Safety Tips: Ensure your lower back remains flat on the ground throughout the movement. Engage your core muscles to avoid straining your back.

Repetitions: 10 reps on each side, 2-3 sets.

Standing Wall Circles (clockwise and counterclockwise)

Objective: To improve shoulder mobility and flexibility.

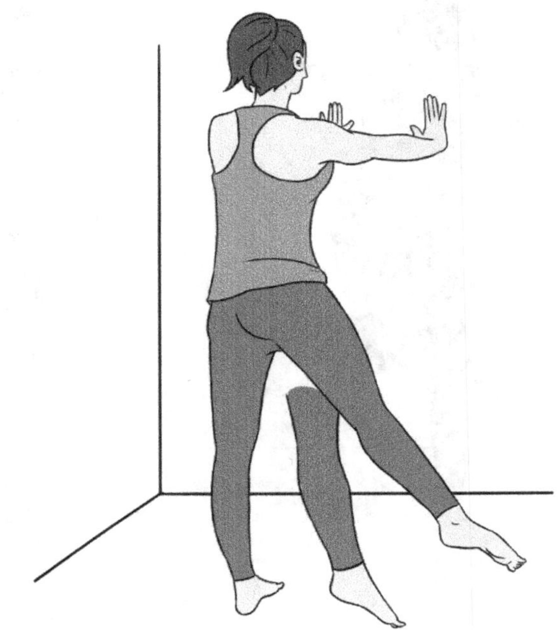

Instructions:

a. Stand with your side to the wall, feet shoulder-width apart.

b. Extend the arm closest to the wall straight out and place your palm on the wall.

c. Slowly make circles with your arm, starting small and gradually increasing the size.

d. After completing the set, repeat the circles in the opposite direction.

e. Switch sides and repeat the exercise with the other arm.

Safety Tips: Keep your spine straight and avoid leaning towards the wall. Make sure the movements are smooth to prevent any jerking motion.

Repetitions: 10 circles in each direction for each arm, 2-3 sets.

Wall Clamshells

Objective: To strengthen the hip muscles and improve hip mobility.

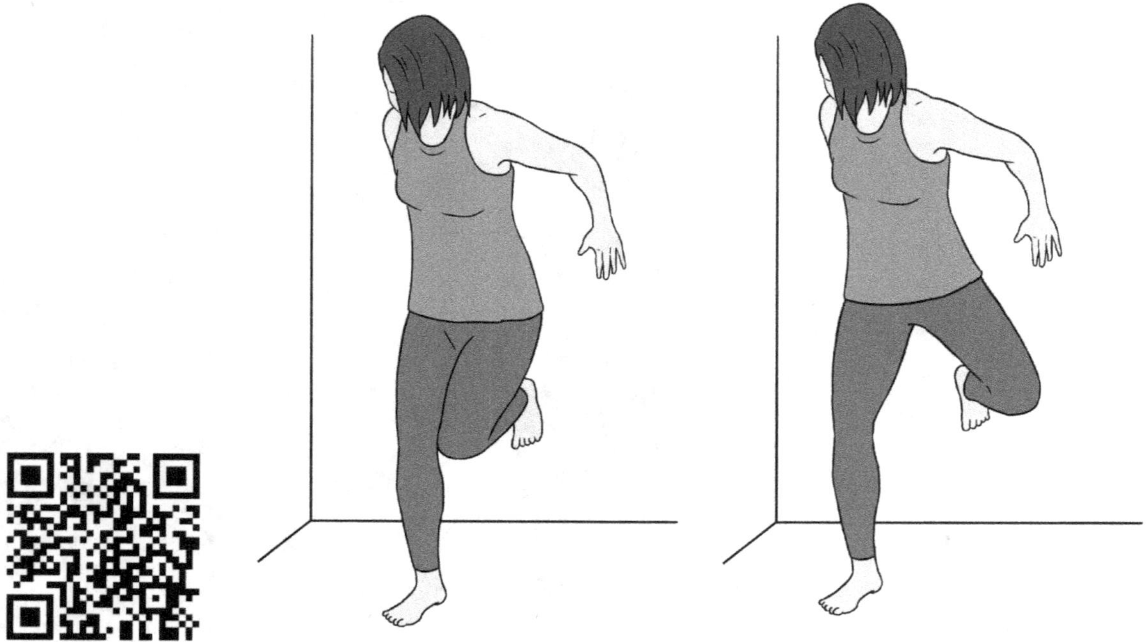

Instructions:

a. Lie on your side with your back against the wall. Your feet, hips, and shoulders should be aligned with the wall.

b. Bend your knees and stack them together, feet touching the wall.

c. Keeping your feet together, lift the top knee as high as you can without moving your bottom knee.

d. Slowly lower the top knee back down to meet the bottom knee.

e. Repeat for the recommended number of repetitions, then switch to the other side.

Safety Tips: Ensure your spine remains neutral and you're not leaning forward or backward. Engage your core to maintain balance.

Repetitions: 15 reps on each side, 2-3 sets.

Wall-assisted Glute Bridges

Objective: To strengthen the glutes, hamstrings, and core.

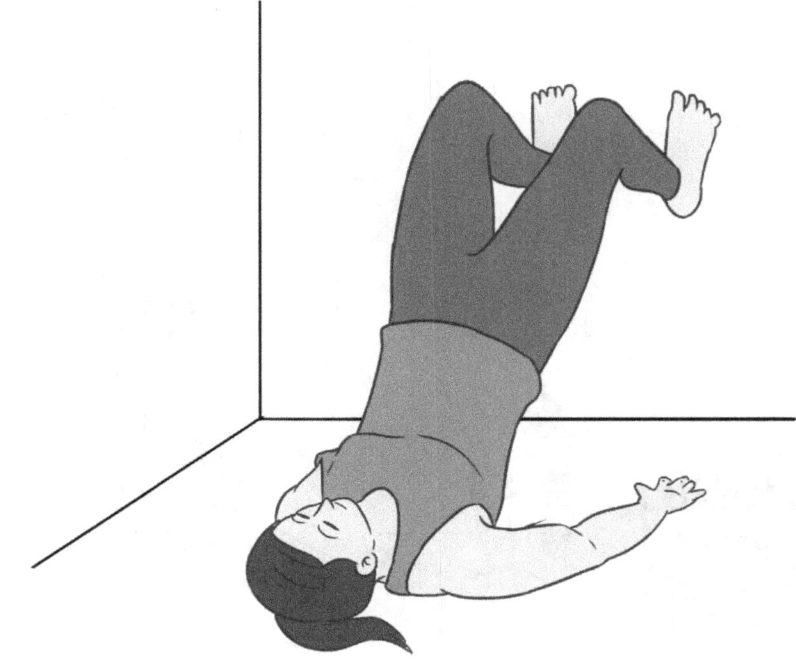

Instructions:

a. Lie on the floor with your feet flat against the wall, knees bent at a 90-degree angle.

b. Arms should be flat on the floor by your side.

c. Pushing through your heels, lift your hips off the ground until your body forms a straight line from your shoulders to your knees.

d. Squeeze your glutes at the top and hold for a moment.

e. Slowly lower your hips back to the starting position. f. Repeat for the recommended number of repetitions.

Safety Tips: Ensure your feet are hip-width apart on the wall and keep your head and shoulders grounded. Avoid over-arching your back.

Repetitions: 12-15 reps, 2-3 sets.

Wall T-push-ups (alternating sides)

Objective: To strengthen the chest, shoulders, and core while improving balance.

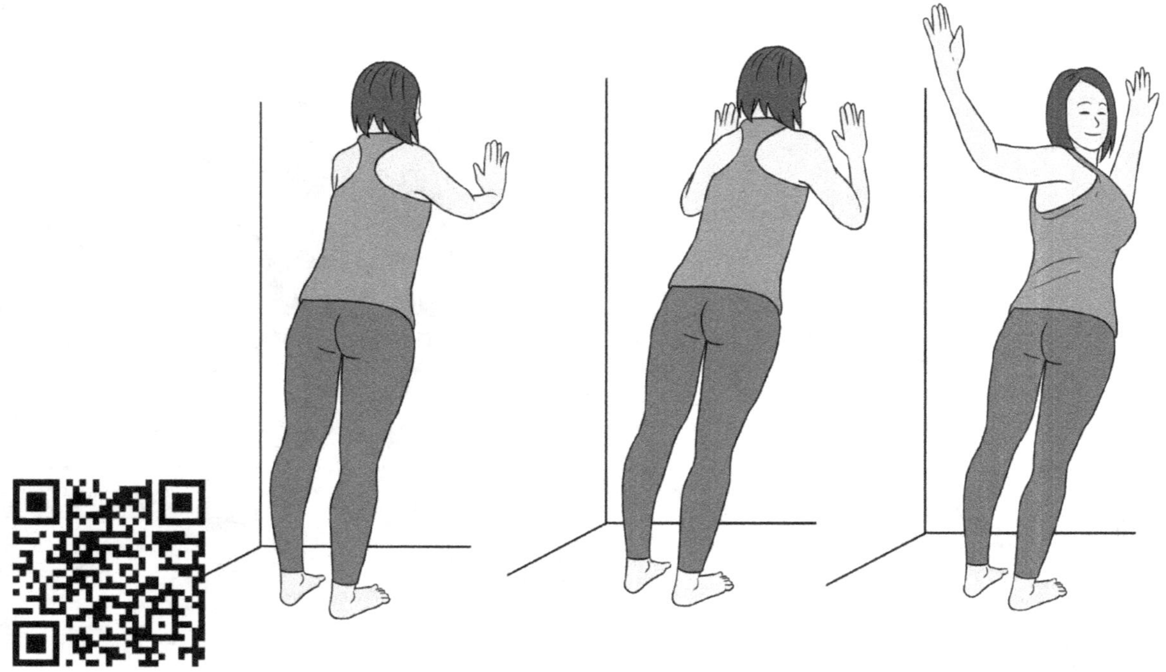

Instructions:

a. Stand arm's length away from the wall, facing it.

b. Place your hands on the wall, wider than shoulder-width apart.

c. Perform a push-up by bending your elbows and leaning your body towards the wall.

d. As you push back, lift your right hand off the wall and rotate your upper body to the right, reaching your right hand towards the ceiling.

e. Return to the starting position and repeat, this time rotating to the left. f. Continue alternating sides for each repetition.

Safety Tips: Keep your body straight from head to heels. Rotate using your core, not just your arm.

Repetitions: 10 reps on each side, 2-3 sets.

Wall-assisted Leg Swings
(front-back and side-side)

Objective: To improve hip mobility and flexibility.

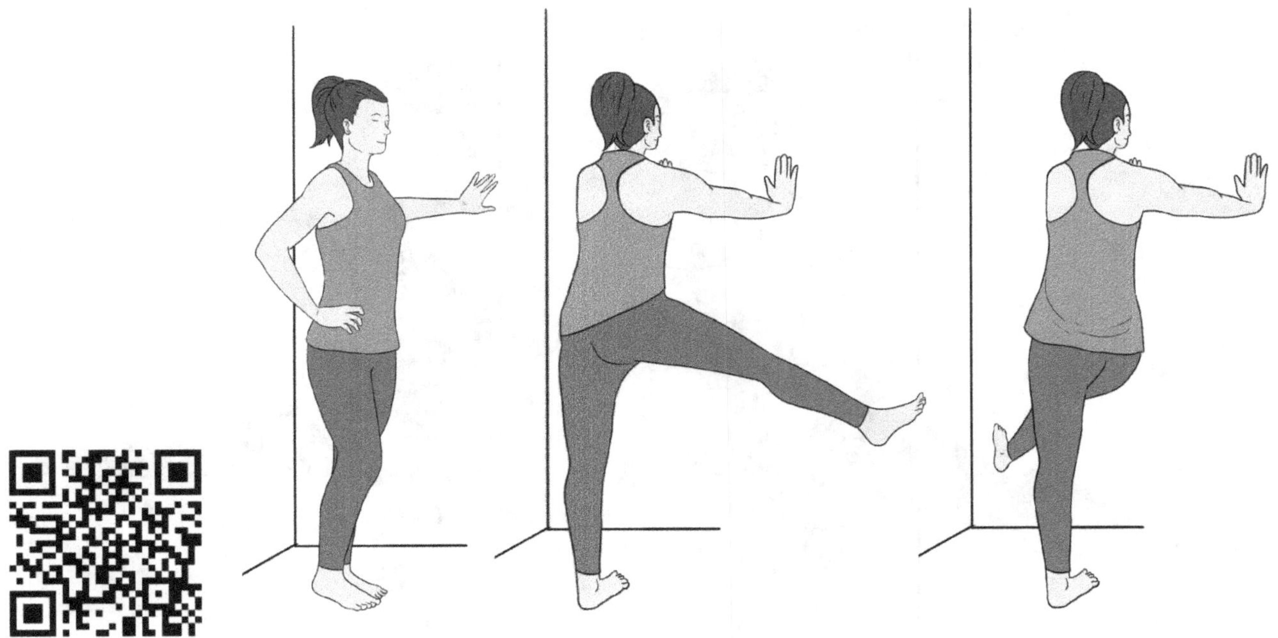

Instructions:

a. Stand next to the wall with your left hand resting on it for support.

b. Keeping your right leg straight, swing it forward and then backward in a controlled motion.

c. After the set, swing the same leg side-to-side in front of your body.

d. Switch to the other leg and repeat.

Safety Tips: Ensure your torso remains upright. Swing your leg only as high as comfortable, avoiding any jerking motions.

Repetitions: 12 swings in each direction for each leg, 2-3 sets.

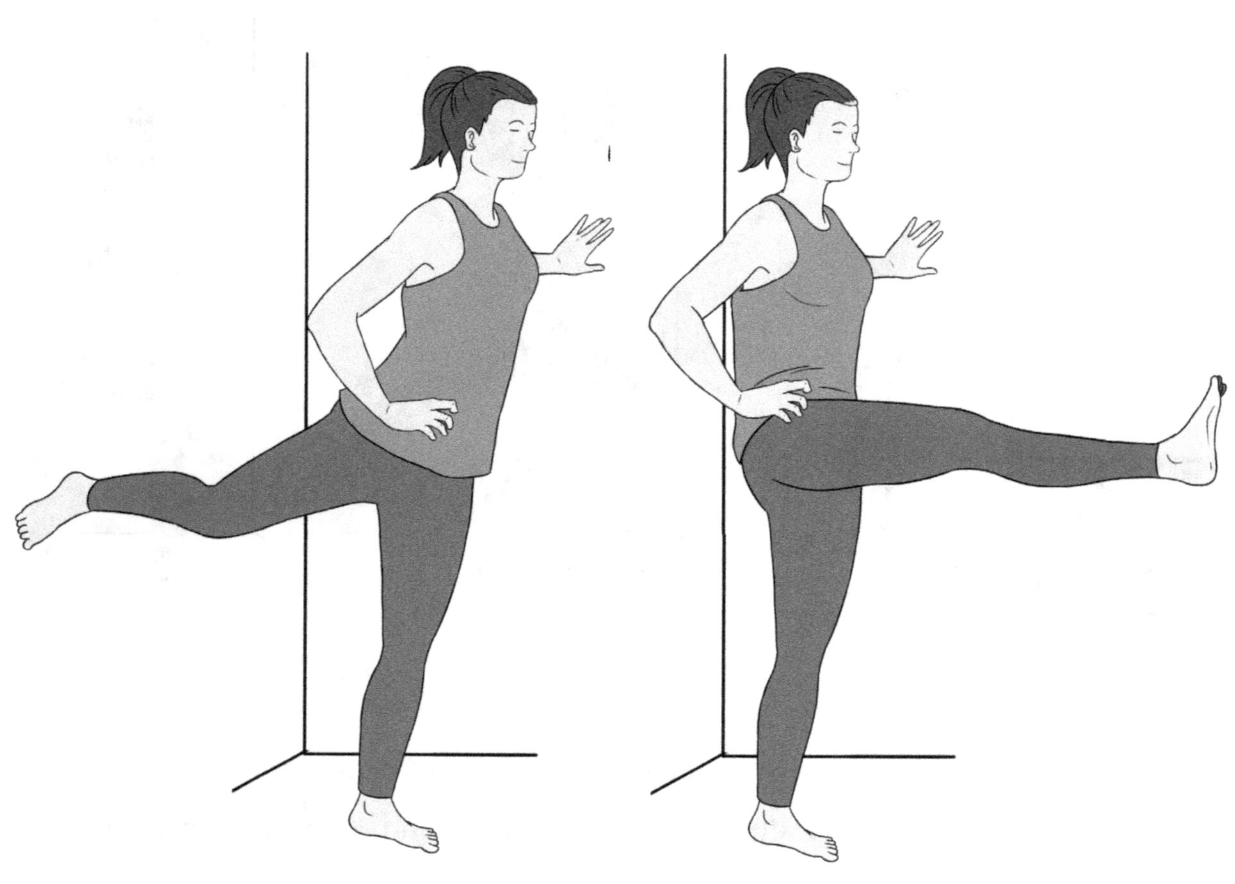

Wall-assisted Seated Spine Stretch

Objective: To stretch and relax the spine, particularly the lower back.

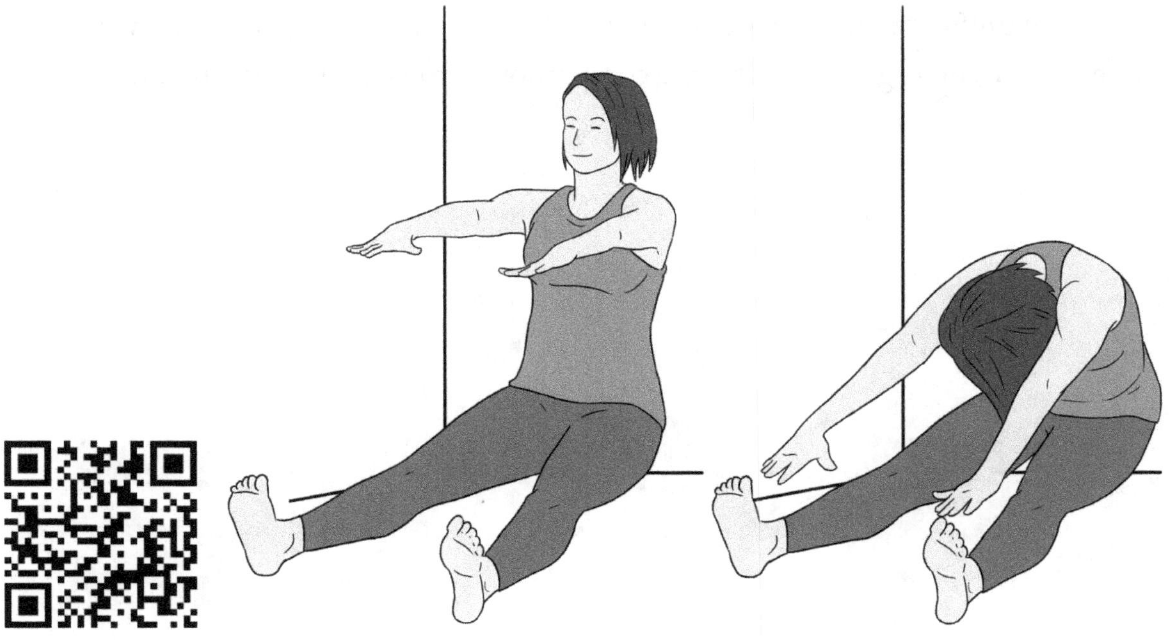

Instructions:

a. Sit on the floor with your back against the wall, legs extended out in front of you.

b. Open your legs wide, feet against the wall.

c. Reach your hands forward between your legs, aiming to touch the floor.

d. Keep your back flat and lean forward, feeling a stretch in your spine and inner thighs.

e. Hold the stretch for a few moments, then sit back up. f. Repeat the stretch for the recommended number of times.

Safety Tips: Ensure you're not rounding your back. Lean forward with a straight spine.

Repetitions: Hold the stretch for 20-30 seconds, 2-3 times.

These exercises, while seeming straightforward, are potent tools in the Wall Pilates toolkit. They engage various muscle groups, ensuring a balanced workout that covers strength, flexibility, and balance. Regular practice of these movements can lead to significant improvements in overall fitness and well-being. The wall, often overlooked, emerges as a versatile companion in the quest for health and vitality.

Chapter 9
Leveling Up: Intermediate Exercises

As with any form of exercise, progression is essential in Wall Pilates. Once the body adapts to foundational movements, it's time to introduce new challenges. This ensures continuous growth, both in strength and flexibility. The intermediate exercises in this chapter offer that next level of challenge. They demand more from the muscles, require better balance, and test endurance. But with consistent practice, these exercises can become a staple in any Wall Pilates routine.

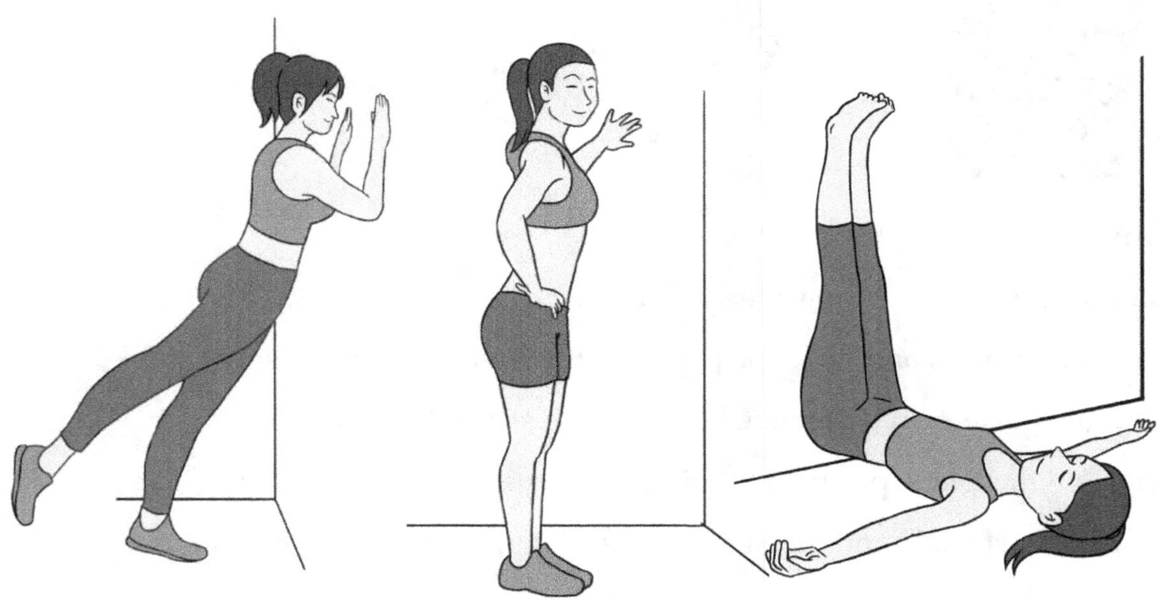

Let's Plank, But on the Wall!

Objective: Strengthen the core, shoulders, and chest.

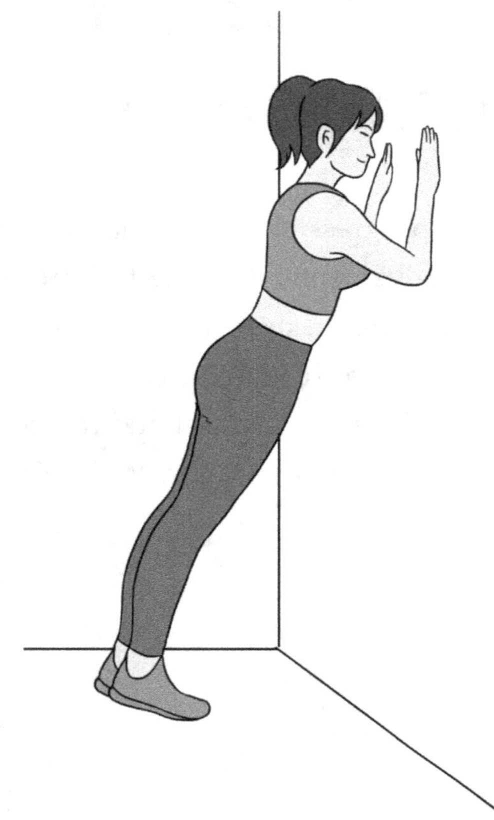

Instructions:

a. Face the wall, standing a few feet away.

b. Lean forward and place the palms on the wall, arms extended.

c. Walk the feet back until the body forms a straight line from head to heels.

d. Hold this plank position, keeping the core engaged and body straight.

e. Breathe steadily and maintain the position for the recommended duration.

Safety Tips: Ensure wrists are below the shoulders. Keep the neck neutral.

Repetitions: Hold for 20-30 seconds, 3 rounds.

Single-Leg Wall Squats

Objective: Strengthen the thighs, glutes, and challenge balance.

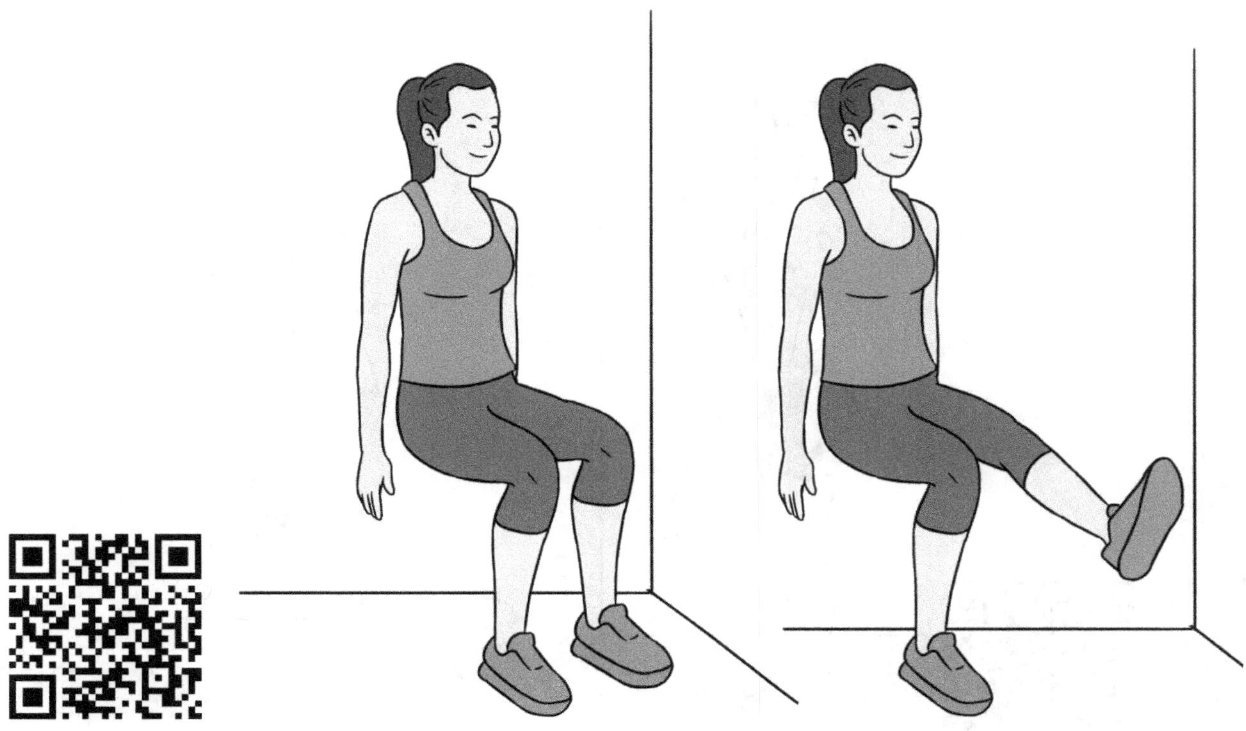

Instructions:

a. Stand with the back against the wall.

b. Lift one foot off the ground, keeping the knee bent.

c. Slowly slide down the wall with the standing leg, as if sitting on an invisible chair.

d. Push through the foot to return to the starting position.

e. Switch legs and repeat.

Safety Tips: Keep the raised foot close to the standing leg. Ensure the knee of the standing leg doesn't extend past the toes.

Repetitions: 8-10 reps on each leg, 2 sets.

Lunge Your Way to Greatness

Objective: Strengthen the thighs, glutes, and improve lower body flexibility.

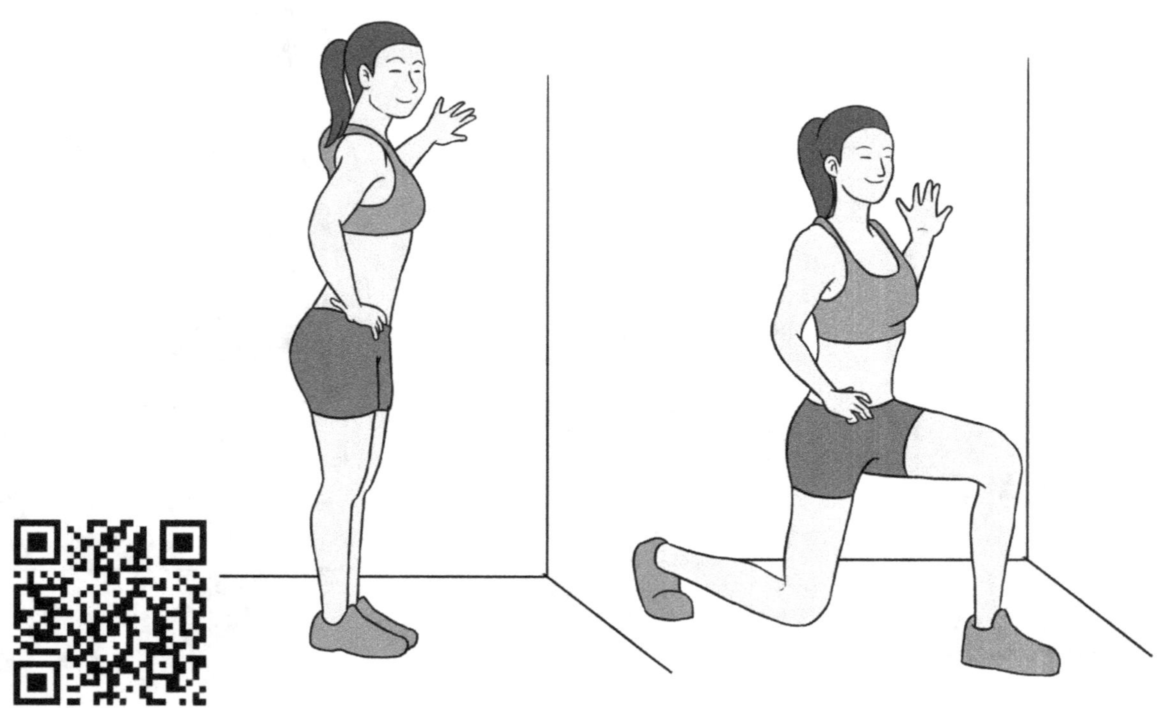

Instructions:

a. Stand facing away from the wall, a couple of feet away.

b. Place the ball of one foot against the wall, leg extended behind.

c. Bend both knees to lower into a lunge, ensuring the front knee is directly above the ankle.

d. Push through the front foot to rise back up.

e. Switch legs and repeat.

Safety Tips: Keep the chest up and shoulders back. Avoid leaning forward.

Repetitions: 8-10 reps on each leg, 2 sets.

Wall Tricep Dips

Objective: Strengthen the triceps and improve upper body stability.

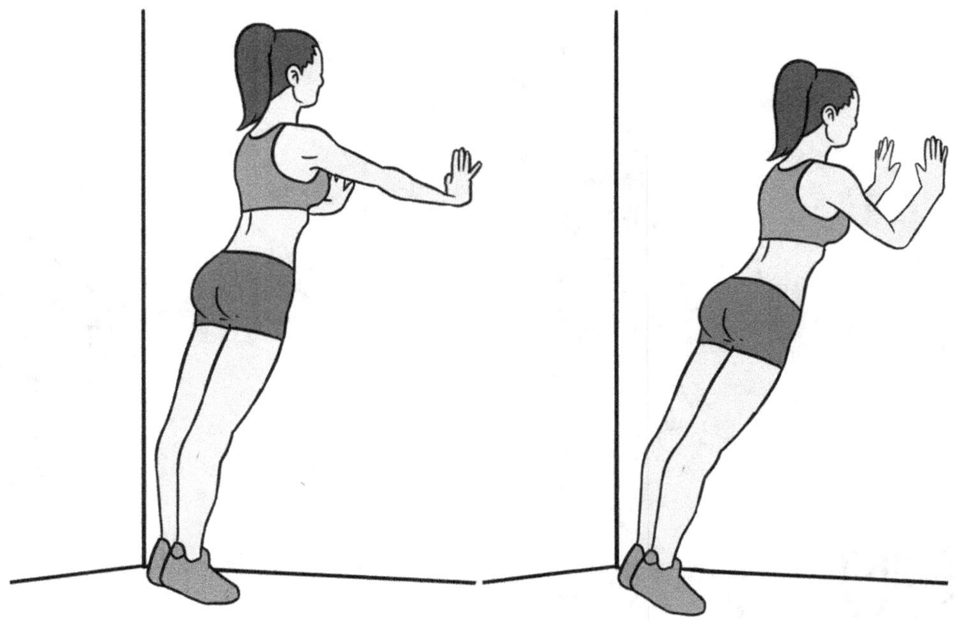

Instructions:

a. Stand two feet away from the wall, adjusting for height.

b. Place hands on the wall behind, at hip height, fingers pointing down or towards you.

c. Lean into the wall with knees slightly bent for stability.

d. Bend elbows to lower your body towards the wall, keeping elbows straight back.

e. Press through palms to extend elbows and return to starting stance, engaging triceps.

Perform 2-3 sets of 8-12 repetitions.

Safety Tips: Keep the elbows pointing straight back. Engage the core.

Wall-assisted Superman Raises

Objective: Strengthen the back, glutes, and shoulders.

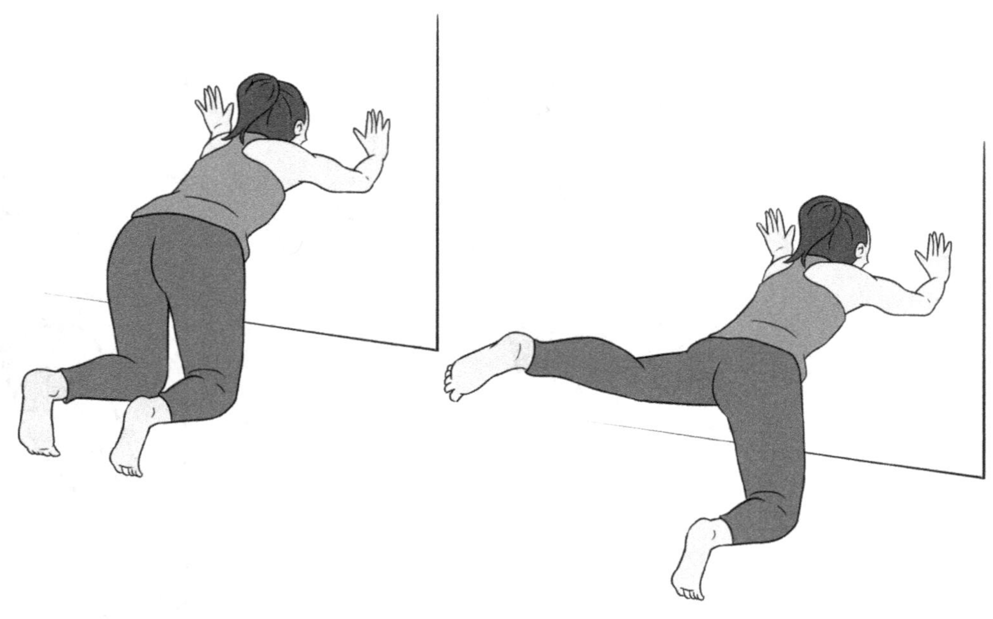

Instructions:

a. Stand facing the wall, a couple of feet away.

b. Lean forward and place both palms on the wall.

c. Keeping one foot on the ground, lift the other leg behind while raising the opposite arm in front.

d. Hold this position briefly, then switch to the other side.

e. Continue alternating for the recommended number of repetitions.

Safety Tips: Keep the back straight and avoid arching. Lift the leg and arm to a comfortable height.

Repetitions: 10 raises on each side, 2 sets.

Wall-assisted Arabesque

Objective: Improve balance, strengthen the glutes, and challenge the core.

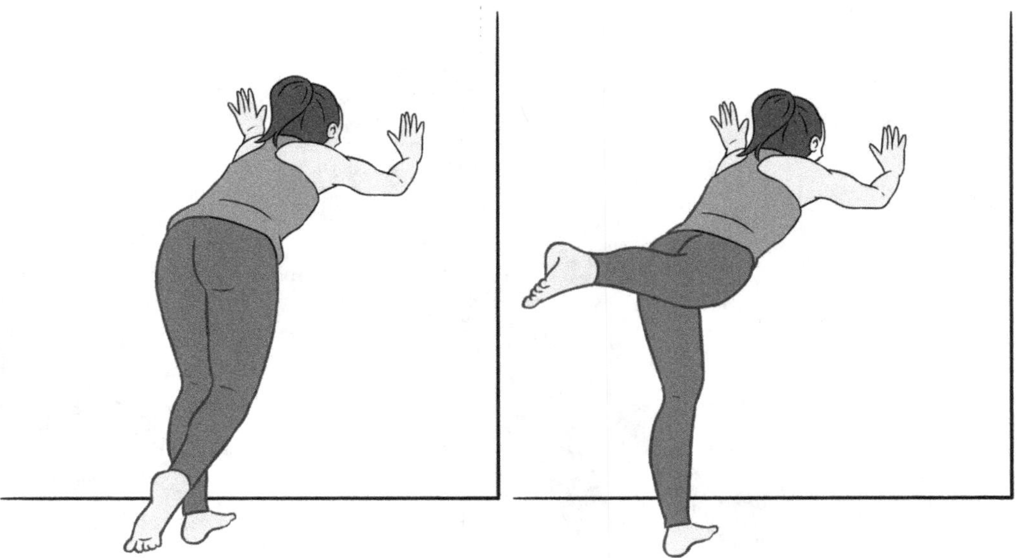

Instructions:

a. Stand a couple of feet away from the wall, facing it.

b. Extend one arm to touch the wall for balance.

c. Shift weight to one foot and slowly lift the other leg behind, keeping it straight.

d. Tilt the upper body forward but keep the back straight.

e. Hold for a few breaths, then return to the starting position. f. Switch sides and repeat.

Safety Tips: Keep the core engaged. Avoid arching the back or tilting the pelvis.

Repetitions: Hold for 10-15 seconds on each side, 3 rounds.

Wall Plank with Alternate Leg Lifts

Objective: Strengthen the core, glutes, and shoulders while improving balance.

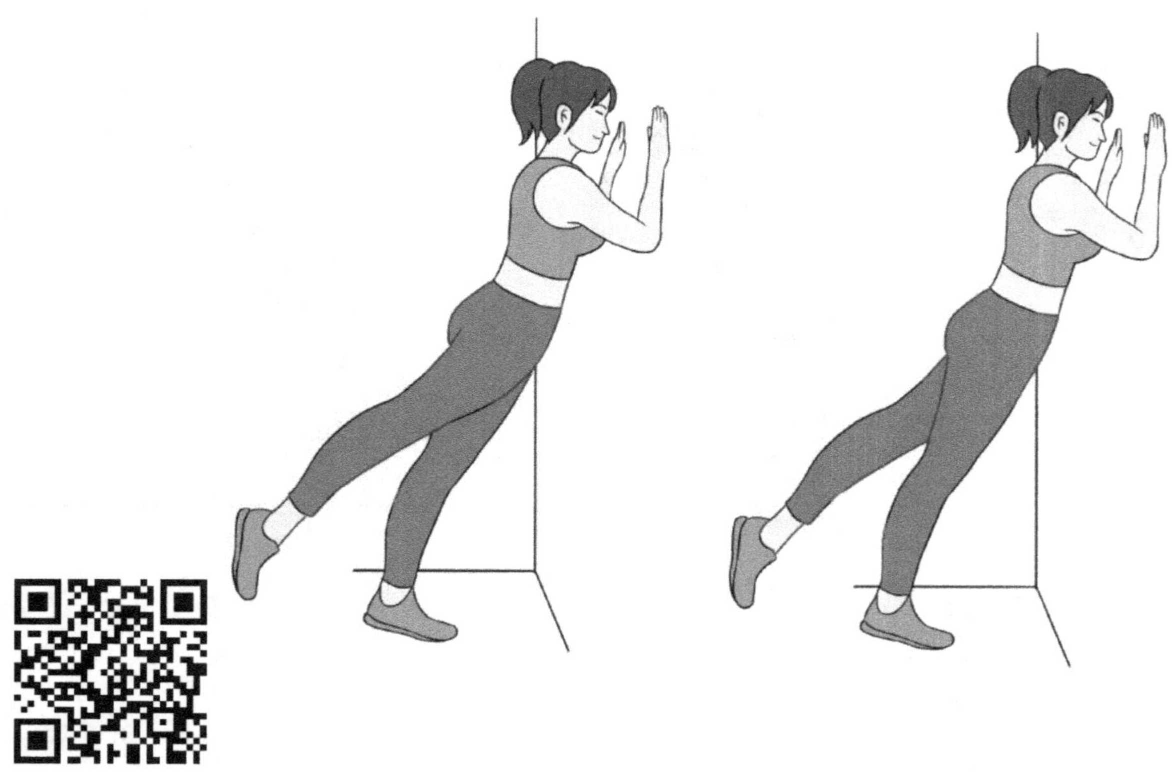

Instructions:

a. Begin in the wall plank position.

b. Keep the core tight and lift one leg up, keeping it straight.

c. Lower the leg back down with control.

d. Lift the other leg and repeat.

e. Continue alternating for the recommended number of repetitions.

Safety Tips: Maintain a straight line from head to heels. Ensure wrists are under the shoulders.

Repetitions: 10 lifts on each leg, 2 sets.

Wall-assisted Scissors

Objective: Strengthen the lower abdominals and improve hip flexibility.

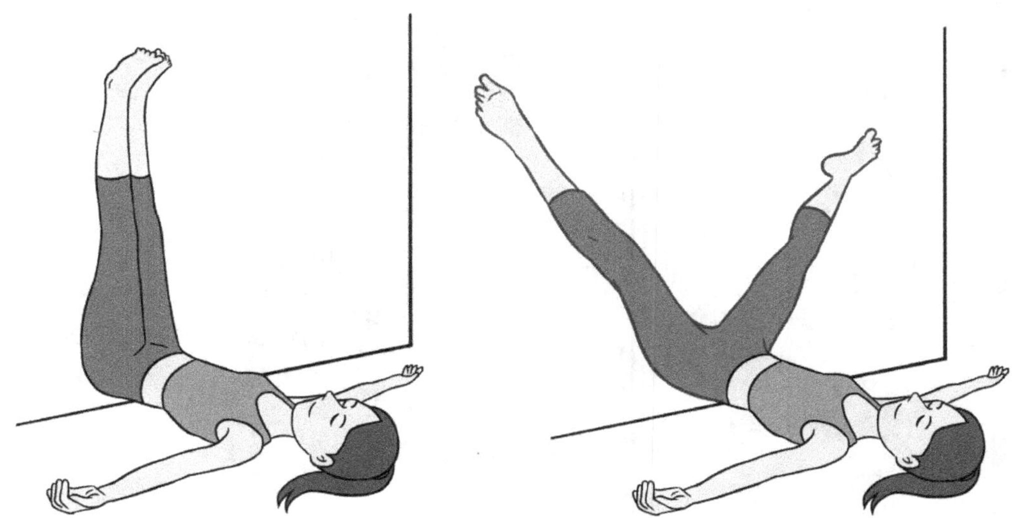

Instructions:

a. Lie on the back with legs lifted and feet pressed against the wall.

b. Keeping one leg on the wall, lower the other leg towards the ground.

c. Lift the lowered leg back up and switch to the other leg.

d. Continue alternating in a scissor-like motion for the recommended number of repetitions.

Safety Tips: Keep the lower back pressed to the floor. Engage the core throughout.

Repetitions: 10 scissors on each leg, 2 sets.

Wall Side Plank (both sides)

Objective: Strengthen the obliques, shoulders, and hips.

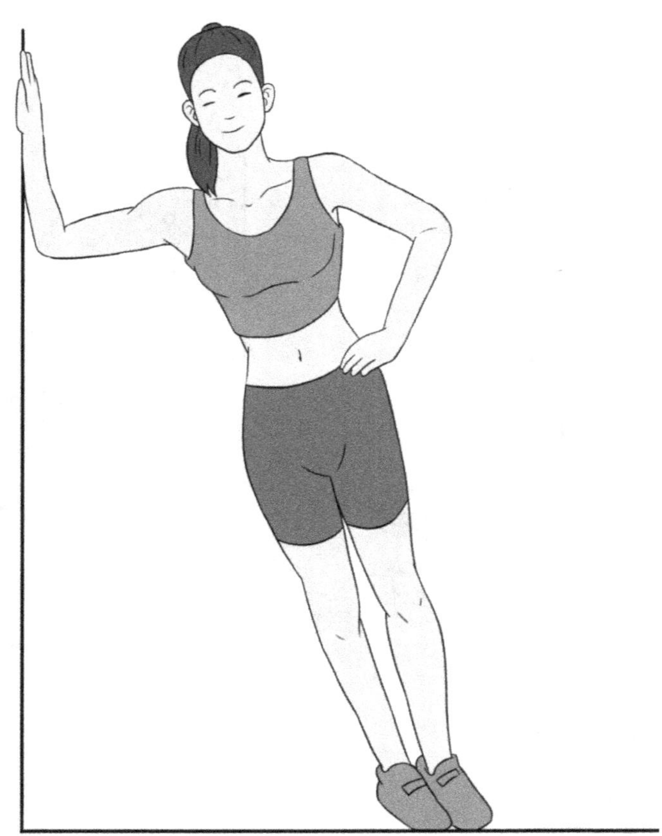

Instructions:

a. Begin by lying on one side, facing perpendicular to the wall.

b. Place the palm of the bottom arm on the floor and the sole of the top foot against the wall.

c. Lift the hips off the ground, pressing through the bottom arm.

d. Hold this side plank position for a few breaths.

e. Lower down and switch sides.

Safety Tips: Stack the feet if not using the wall for support. Keep the body in a straight line.

Repetitions: Hold for 20-25 seconds on each side, 3 rounds.

Wall-assisted Spinal Rotation Stretch

Objective: Improve spine flexibility and relieve tension in the back.

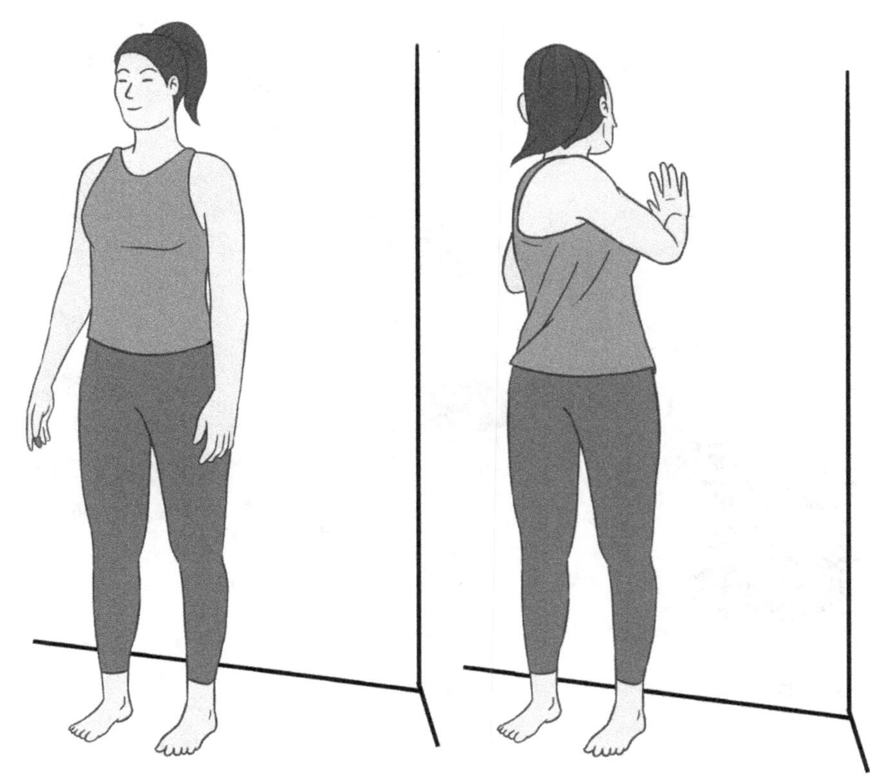

Instructions:

a. Sit on the floor with the right side of the body next to the wall, knees bent.

b. Twist the upper body to the left and place both palms on the wall.

c. Gently push against the wall to deepen the twist.

d. Hold for a few breaths, then switch sides and repeat.

Safety Tips: Rotate from the waist, not the lower back. Keep the spine long.

Repetitions: Hold for 20-30 seconds on each side, 2 rounds.

Wall-assisted Plank to Pike

Objective: To challenge the core, shoulders, and upper back.

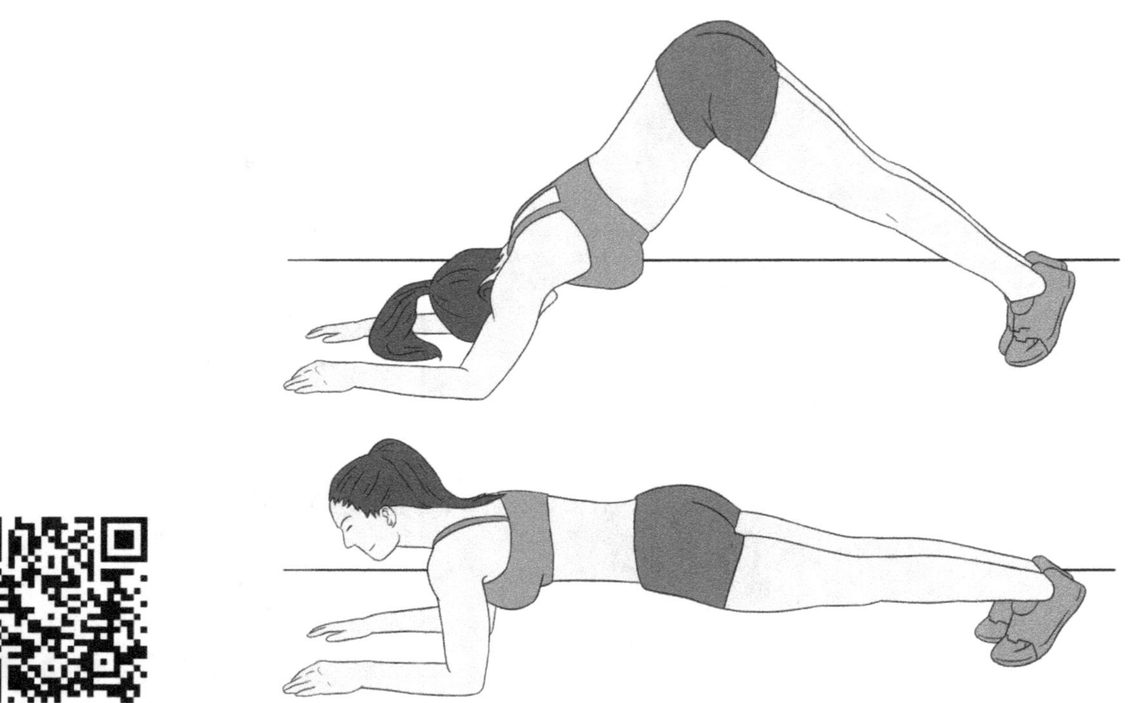

Instructions:

a. Start by facing away from the wall in a plank position, with your feet resting on the base of the wall.

b. Ensure your body forms a straight line from your head to your heels.

c. Slowly walk your feet up the wall while pushing your hips upwards, forming an inverted V or a pike position.

d. Hold for a moment at the top, then slowly return to the plank position.

e. Repeat for the recommended number of repetitions.

Safety Tips: Keep your hands directly below your shoulders. Engage your core throughout the exercise to support your back.

Repetitions: 8-10 reps, 2-3 sets.

Wall-assisted Reverse Lunges

Objective: To strengthen the quads, hamstrings, glutes, and improve balance.

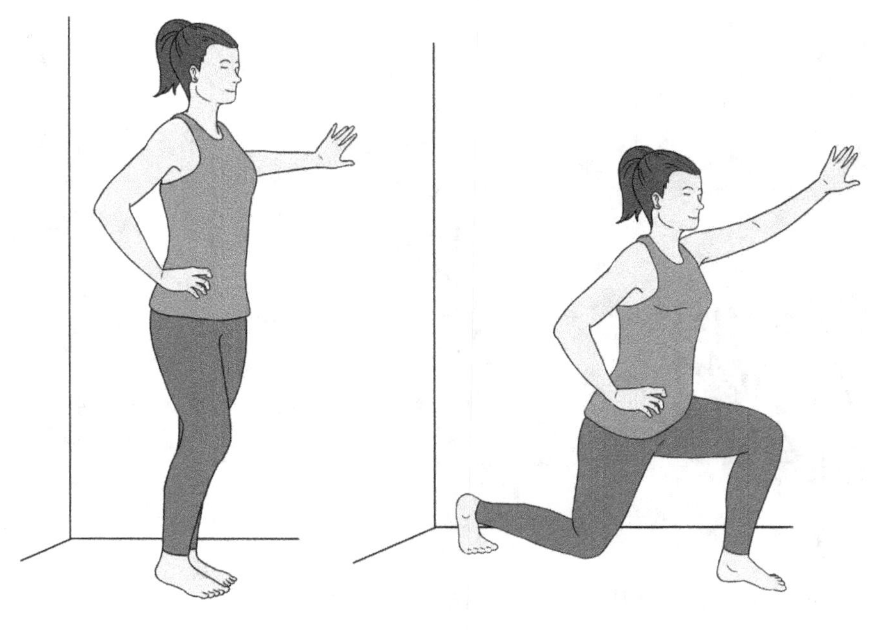

Instructions:

a. Stand facing away from the wall, about two feet away.

b. Place your hands on your hips and stand tall.

c. Step your right foot back and place the ball of the foot on the wall.

d. Bend both knees to lower into a lunge, ensuring your left knee is directly above your left ankle.

e. Press into your left heel to rise back up. f. Complete the set on one leg, then switch to the other.

Safety Tips: Maintain a tall posture throughout. Avoid letting your front knee move past your toes.

Repetitions: 12 reps on each leg, 2-3 sets.

Standing Wall-assisted Torsion Control

Objective: To enhance oblique strength and improve torso rotation control.

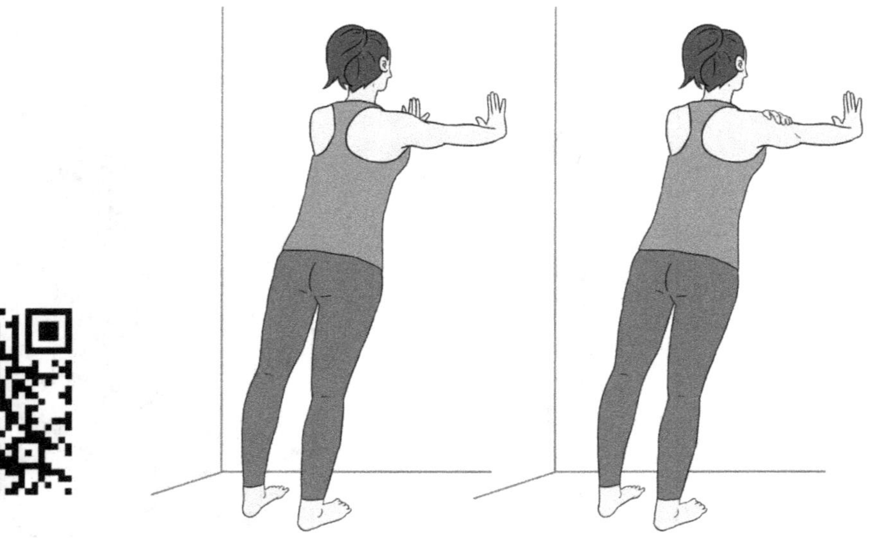

Instructions:

a. Position yourself an arm's length in front of a wall.

b. Stretch your arms out in front of you, palms flat against the wall, keeping your hips facing forward.

c. Twist your upper body towards the wall by lifting one hand off the wall and placing it on the shoulder of the arm still in contact with the wall. Then alternate hands to perform the rotation on both sides.

d. Use the side muscles of your abdomen (obliques) to control the rotation movement.

e. Gradually come back to the initial position with both hands on the wall and repeat for the set number of repetitions.

f. After completing the rotations on one side, switch to the opposite side to ensure balanced muscle engagement.

Safety Tips: Keep your feet hip-width apart and firmly grounded. Ensure the rotation comes from the waist and not the hips.

Repetitions: 10 reps on each side, 2-3 sets.

Wall-assisted Single Leg Deadlift

Objective: To build strength in the hamstrings, glutes, and lower back while also enhancing balance.

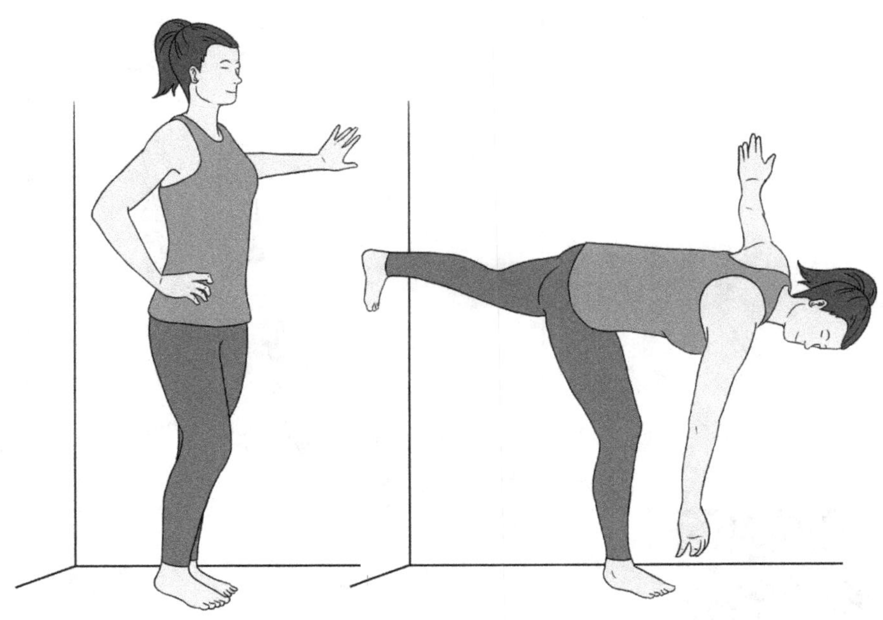

Instructions:

a. Stand beside the wall, about an arm's length away.

b. Lean forward slightly, placing your palm flat against the wall at chest height.

c. Shift your weight onto your left foot.

d. Slowly lift your right leg behind you while hinging at the hips, keeping the leg straight.

e. Lower your chest towards the wall, aiming for a parallel position with the floor.

f. Push through your left foot to return to the starting position. g. Complete the set on one leg, then switch to the other.

Safety Tips: Keep the back straight and the core engaged throughout the movement. Avoid rounding the back.

Repetitions: 10 reps on each leg, 2-3 sets.

Wall-assisted Starfish Sequence

Objective: To work on core strength and stability.

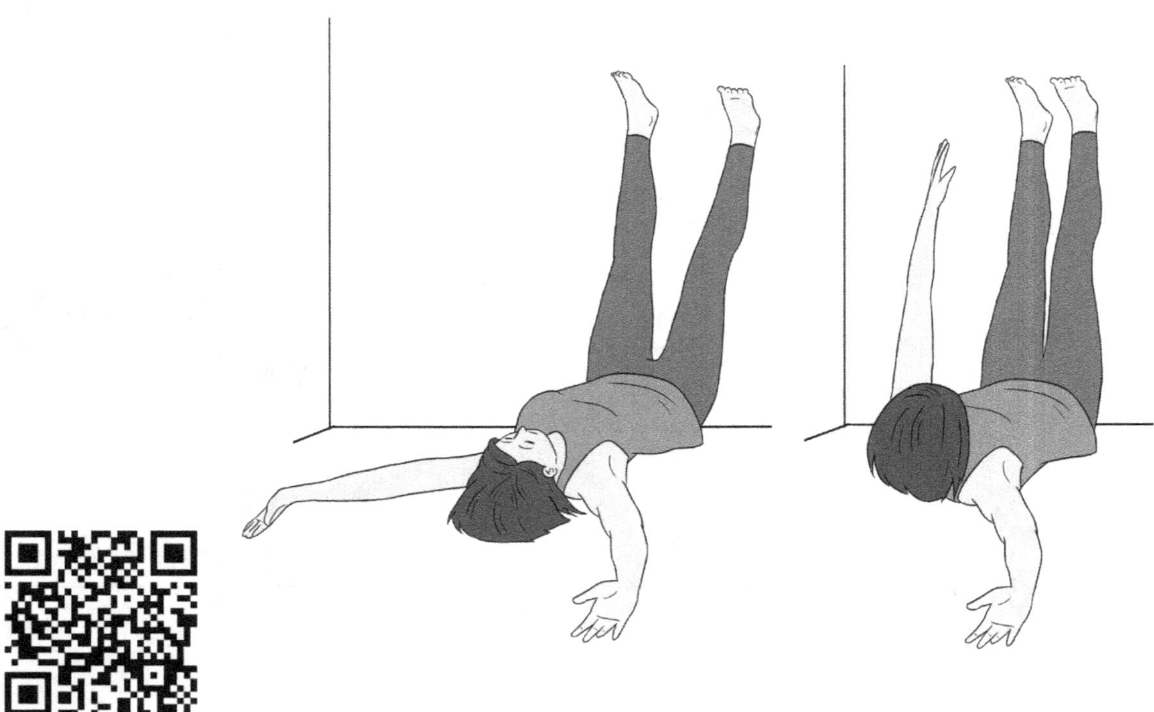

Instructions:

a. Start by lying on the ground, with your legs straight and your feet against the wall.

b. Prop yourself up on your elbow, ensuring it's directly below your shoulder.

c. Lift your hips off the ground to form a straight line from head to heels.

d. Raise your top arm and leg simultaneously, forming a "starfish" shape.

e. Hold for a moment, then lower the arm and leg back down. f. After completing one side, switch to the other.

Safety Tips: Keep the hips lifted and avoid sagging. Engage the core throughout the exercise.

Repetitions: 8 reps on each side, 2-3 sets.

Wall-assisted Jackknife

Objective: To target the abdominal muscles and improve core strength.

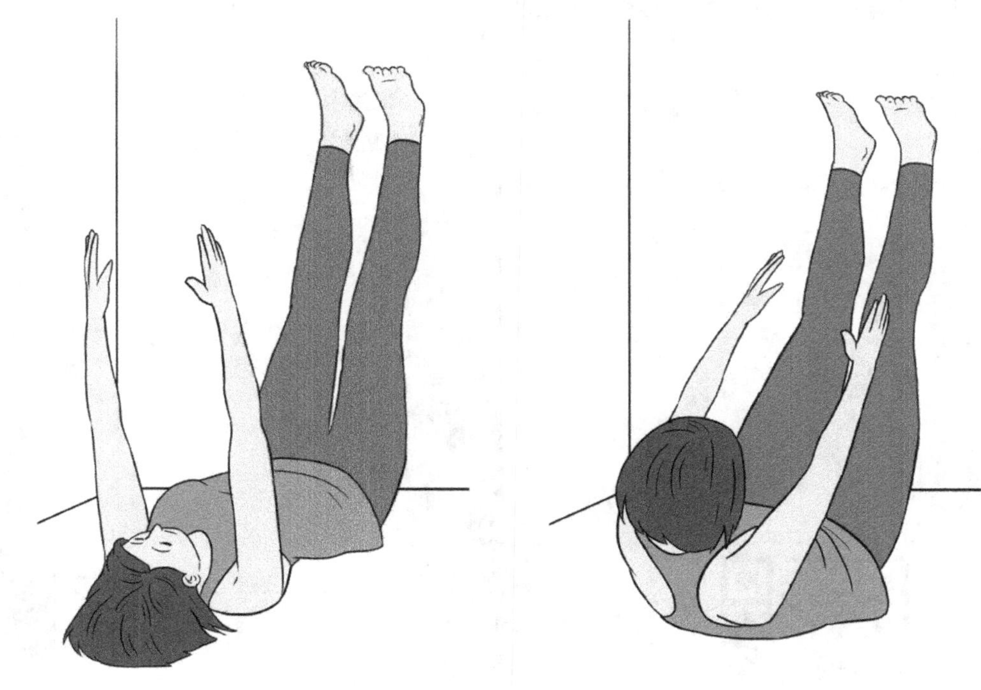

Instructions:

a. Lie on your back with your legs extended upwards and feet flat against the wall.

b. Extend your arms behind your head.

c. In a smooth motion, lift your upper body off the ground, reaching your hands towards your feet.

d. Lower yourself back down with control.

e. Repeat for the recommended number of repetitions.

Safety Tips: Ensure the movement is controlled. Avoid straining the neck by keeping the gaze upwards.

Repetitions: 12-15 reps, 2-3 sets.

Wall Plank Knee to Elbow
(alternating sides)

Objective: To engage the core, shoulders, and obliques.

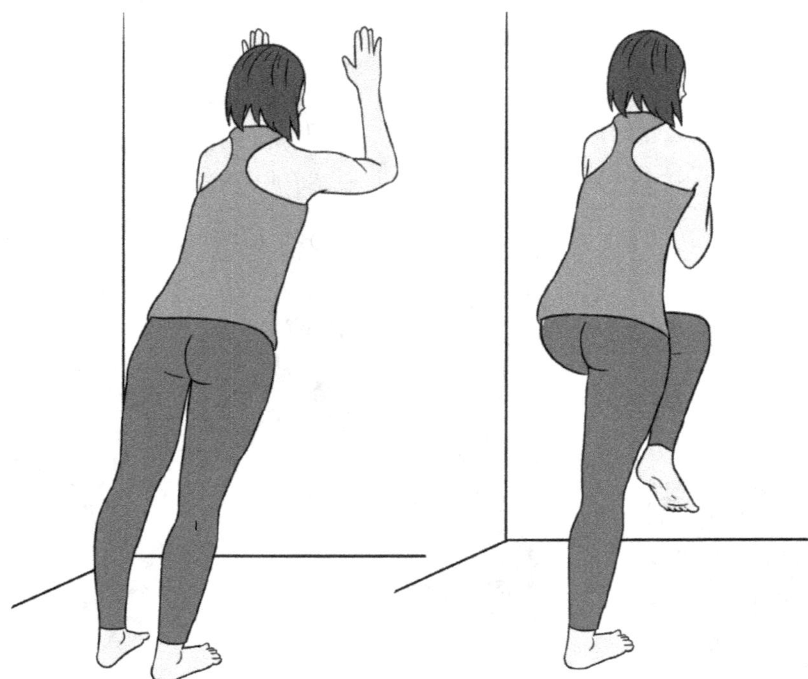

Instructions:

a. Begin in a plank position facing away from the wall, with feet resting against its base.

b. Ensure the body forms a straight line from head to heels.

c. Lift your right knee and bring it towards your left elbow.

d. Return to the starting position.

e. Now, lift your left knee towards your right elbow. f. Continue alternating sides for the set duration.

Safety Tips: Maintain a strong plank position throughout, avoiding any sagging in the hips.

Repetitions: 10 reps on each side, 2-3 sets.

The beauty of Wall Pilates lies in its versatility. Whether someone is a beginner or has been practicing for years, there's always a new movement to try or a familiar one to refine. These intermediate exercises bridge the gap between foundational movements and advanced techniques. They challenge the body in new ways, ensuring that strength, flexibility, and balance continue to improve. The wall, in its quiet support, remains a constant ally, providing stability when needed and offering resistance when desired. With each passing session, the rewards of Wall Pilates become more evident. The body feels stronger, movements become more fluid, and there's a sense of accomplishment that comes from mastering a new set of exercises. The journey with Wall Pilates, supported by the humble wall, is filled with endless possibilities and countless gains.

Chapter 10
For the Brave: Advanced Exercises

The essence of Wall Pilates is its adaptability. It can be as gentle or as challenging as one wishes it to be. But for those who have been consistent, felt the burn, and tasted the sweet progress of moving from beginner to intermediate exercises, there comes a point when the heart yearns for something even more challenging. This chapter is for those brave souls.

These exercises are not just movements; they're a testament to dedication, patience, and the sheer will to push boundaries. They're about tapping into unknown reserves of strength and realizing that the wall, a silent partner so far, can help unlock so much more.

Mountain Climbers, Wall-Style

Objective: Strengthen the core, boost cardiovascular health, and improve leg power.

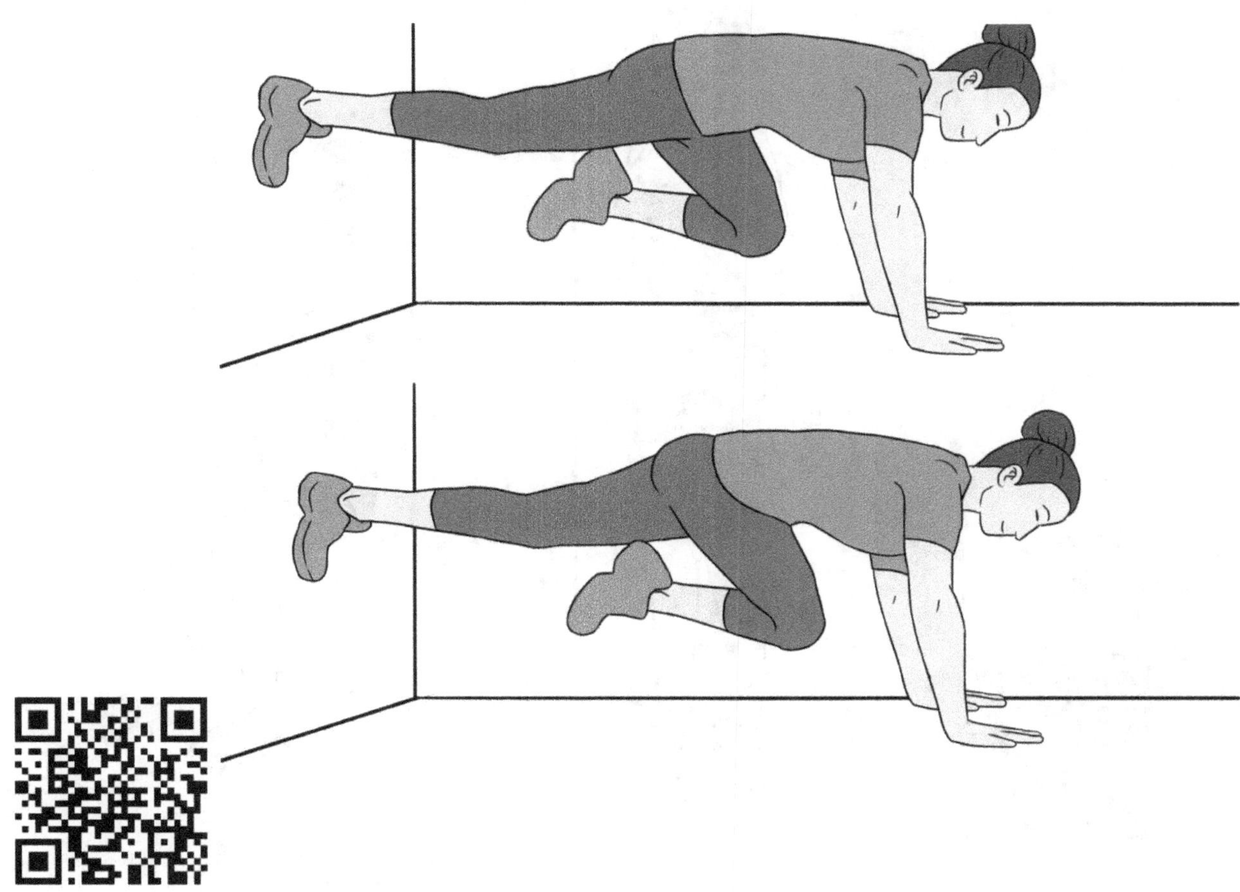

Instructions:

a. Begin in a plank position with feet against the wall.

b. Drive one knee towards the chest, then quickly switch to the other leg.

c. Continue the motion, alternating legs, while maintaining a strong plank form.

Safety Tips: Keep the body in a straight line. Don't let the hips sag.

Repetitions: 20-25 reps on each leg, 2 sets.

The Art of the Isometric Wall Sit

Objective: Strengthen the quadriceps and build endurance.

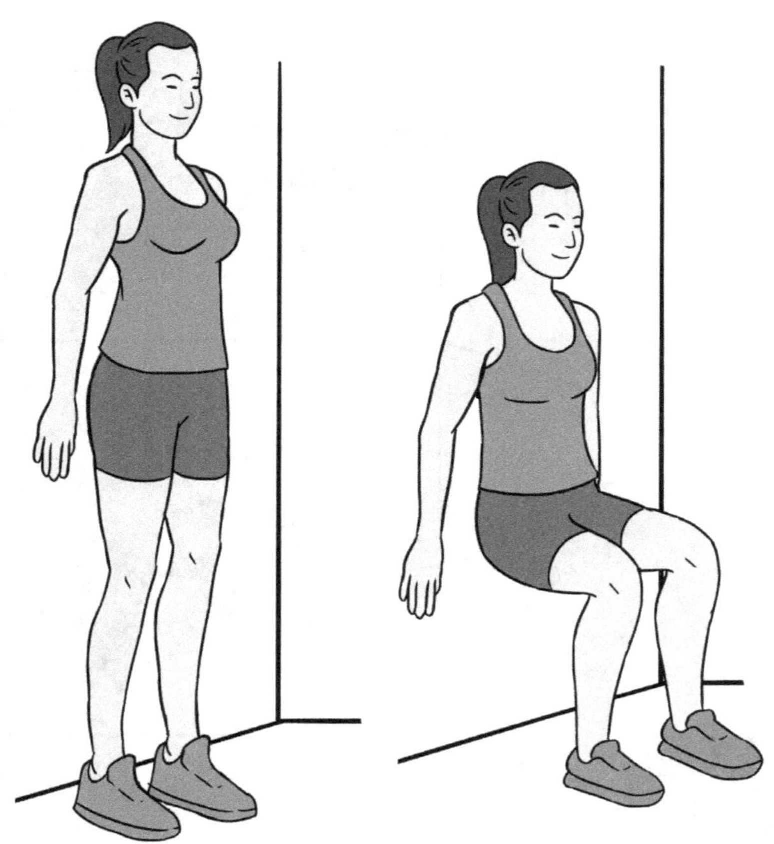

Instructions:

a. Stand with back against the wall.

b. Slide down into a seated position, knees bent at 90 degrees.

c. Hold the position, keeping the back flat against the wall.

Safety Tips: Ensure knees are directly above ankles, not pushing out over the toes.

Repetitions: Hold for 30-60 seconds, 3 rounds.

Wall Handstands (Partial)

Objective: Strengthen the shoulders, arms, and core. Improve balance.

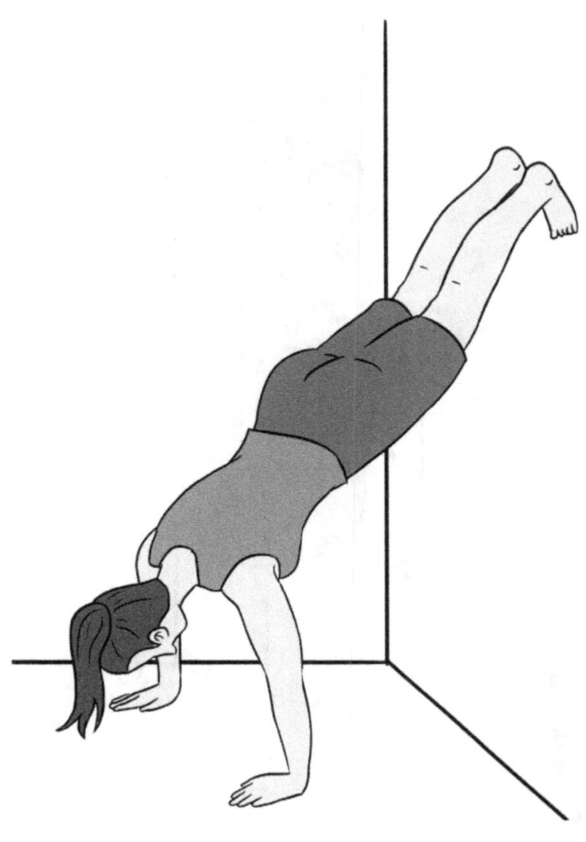

Instructions:

a. Start facing the wall, hands on the ground.

b. Kick one leg up, followed by the other, so both feet are resting on the wall.

c. Hold the position, aiming to get the body in a straight line.

Safety Tips: Keep the core engaged. Push through the palms to lift the body upwards.

Repetitions: Hold for 10-15 seconds, 2-3 attempts.

Advanced Wall Squat with Alternate Leg Lifts

Objective: Strengthen the quadriceps, glutes, and core. Improve balance.

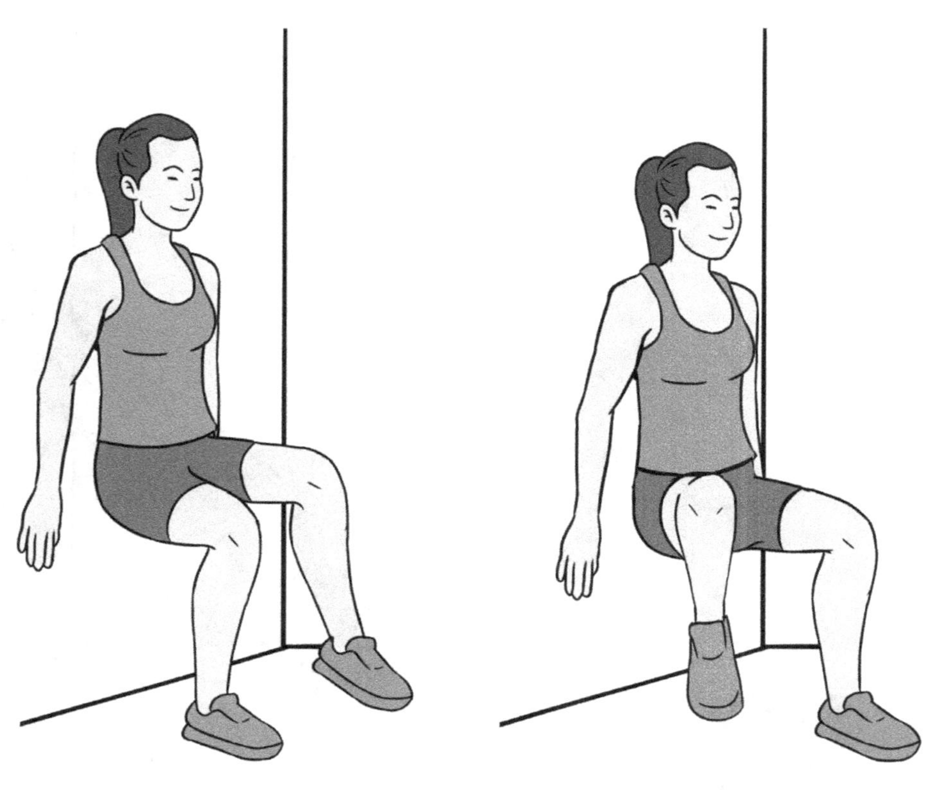

Instructions:

a. Begin in the wall sit position.

b. Lift one leg off the ground, keeping it straight.

c. Lower it with control, then lift the other leg.

d. Continue alternating for the recommended number of reps.

Safety Tips: Keep the back pressed to the wall. Engage the core throughout.

Repetitions: 10-12 lifts on each leg, 2 sets.

Wall Walks (starting in a plank and walking feet up the wall)

Objective: Improve upper body strength, especially in the shoulders. Enhance core stability.

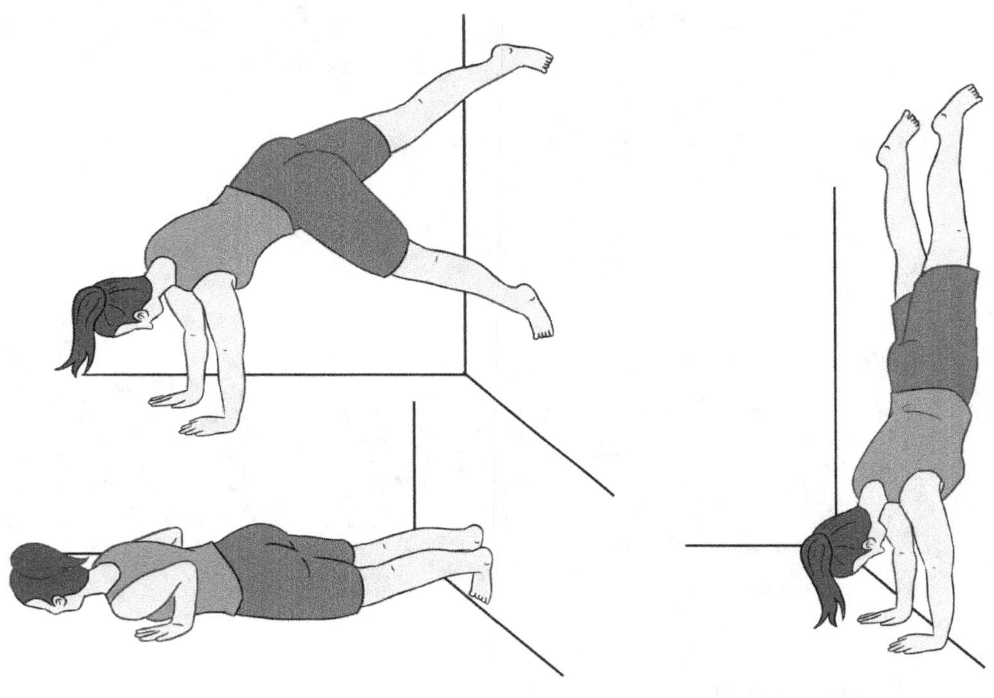

Instructions:

a. Start in a plank position with feet close to the wall.

b. Begin walking the feet up the wall while moving the hands closer.

c. Walk as high as comfort allows, then slowly walk back down to the starting position.

Safety Tips: Move with control. Keep the body in a straight line as it moves.

Repetitions: 4-5 wall walks, 2 sets.

Wall-assisted Roll-Ups

Objective: Strengthen the core, especially the abdominal muscles, and increase flexibility in the spine.

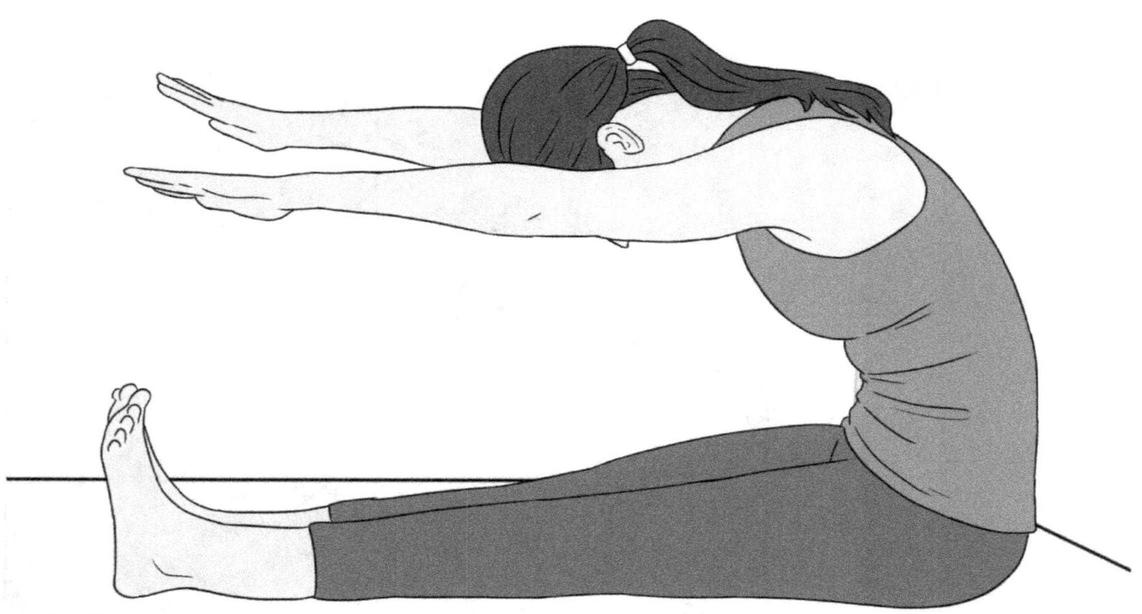

Instructions:
a. Start seated with legs extended in front and back flat against the wall.
b. Inhale deeply. On the exhale, slowly roll down one vertebra at a time, keeping the spine pressed against the wall.
c. Once lying flat, inhale again. On the next exhale, lift the head and shoulders and roll back up to the seated position.
Safety Tips: Keep movements slow and controlled. Ensure the spine moves segment by segment.
Repetitions: 8-10 roll-ups, 2 sets.

Single-Leg Wall Plank with Pulse

Objective: Strengthen the core, glutes, and shoulders, while improving balance.

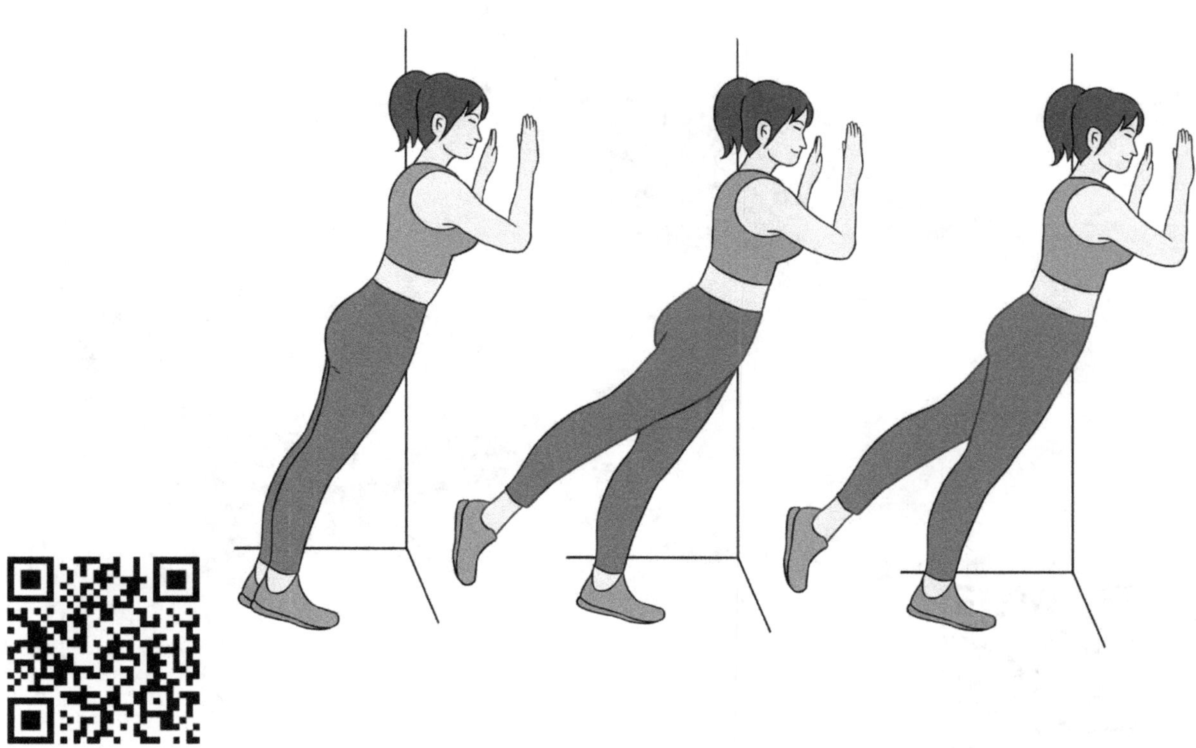

Instructions:

a. Start in a plank position with feet against the wall.

b. Lift one leg off the wall, keeping it straight.

c. Pulse the lifted leg up and down in a small, controlled motion.

d. Switch legs and repeat.

Safety Tips: Maintain a strong plank form throughout. Engage the glutes during the leg pulse.

Repetitions: 10-12 pulses on each leg, 2 sets.

Wall-assisted Swan Dive

Objective: Strengthen the back muscles and open up the chest, promoting better posture.

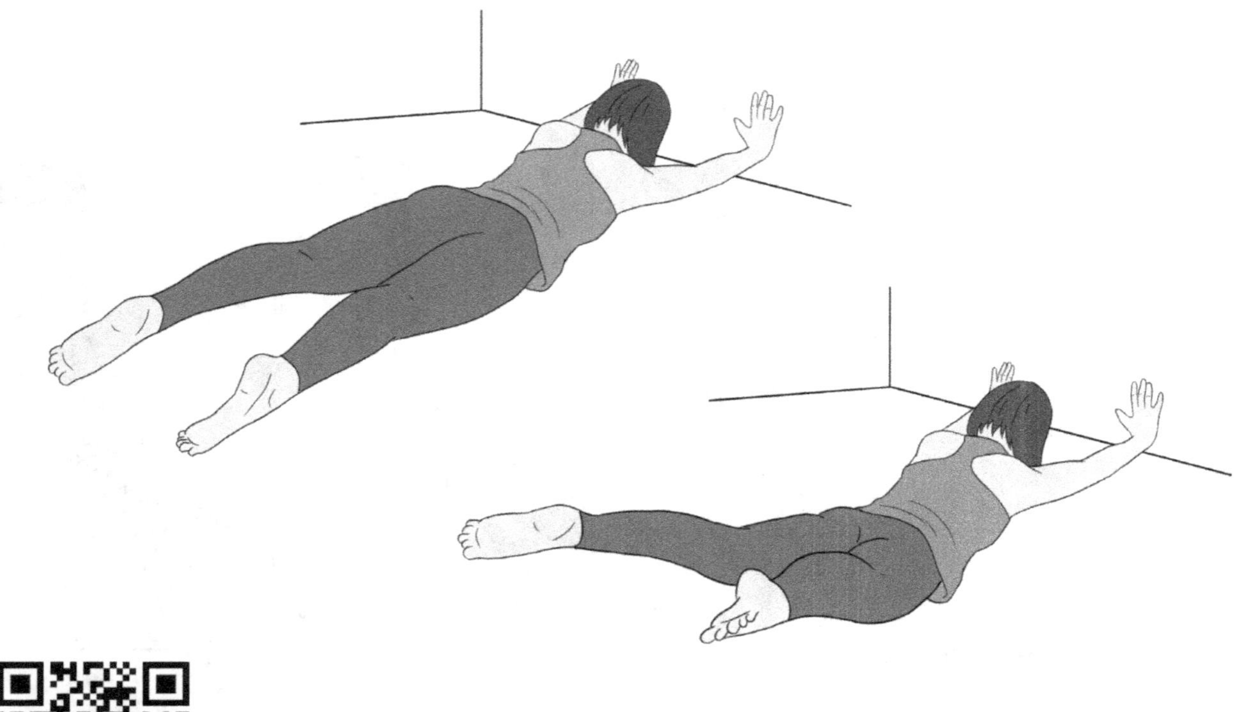

Instructions:

a. Stand facing away from the wall, a couple of feet away.

b. Hinge at the hips and lean forward with arms extended behind, fingertips touching the wall.

c. Use the wall for support as you lift the chest and arch the back, diving forward, and then returning to the starting position.

Safety Tips: Keep movements smooth and avoid any jerky motions. Ensure the lower back doesn't strain.

Repetitions: 6-8 dives, 2 sets.

Wall Plank with Rotation

Objective: Enhance core stability and strengthen the obliques.

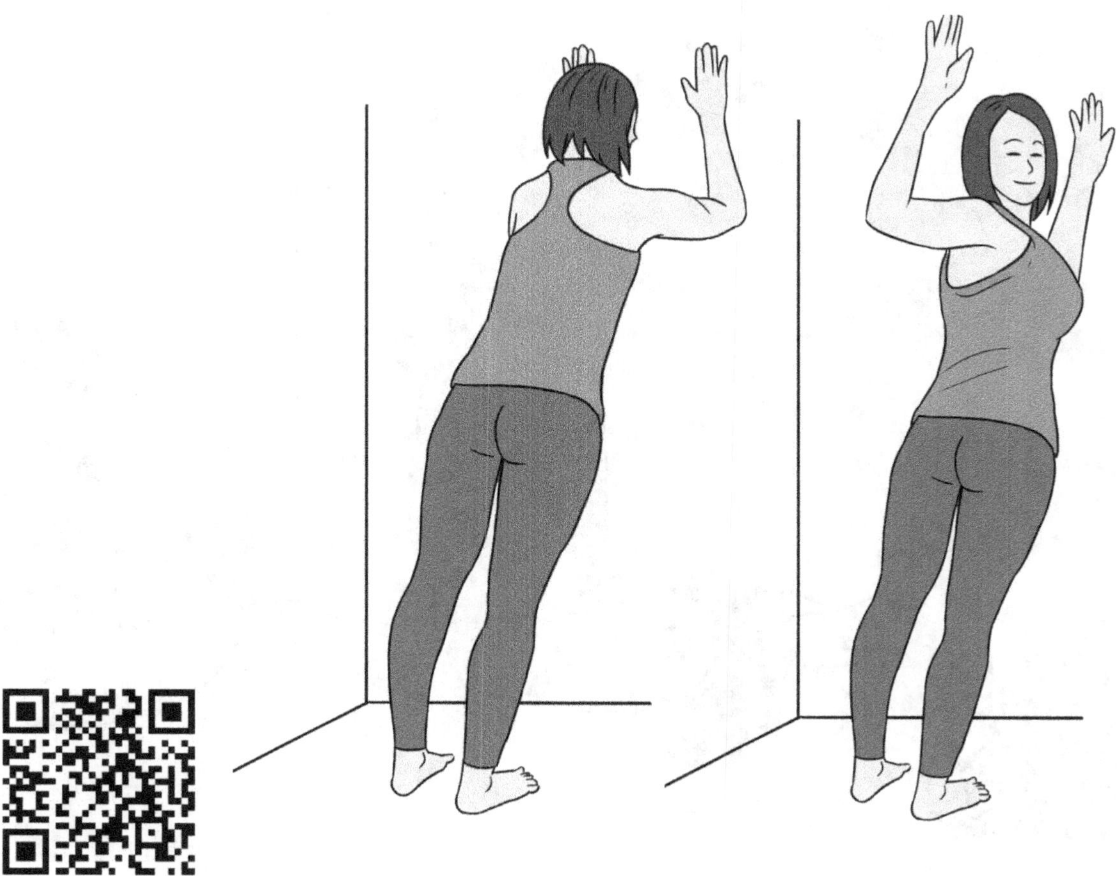

Instructions:

a. Begin in a side plank position with one hand on the ground and feet against the wall.

b. Lift the top arm, then rotate the torso and thread the top arm under the body.

c. Return to the side plank and repeat.

Safety Tips: Keep the body in a straight line during the rotation. Engage the core to ensure stability.

Repetitions: 8-10 rotations on each side, 2 sets.

Wall-assisted Criss-Cross (Pilates Bicycle)

Objective: Strengthen the obliques and improve core stability.

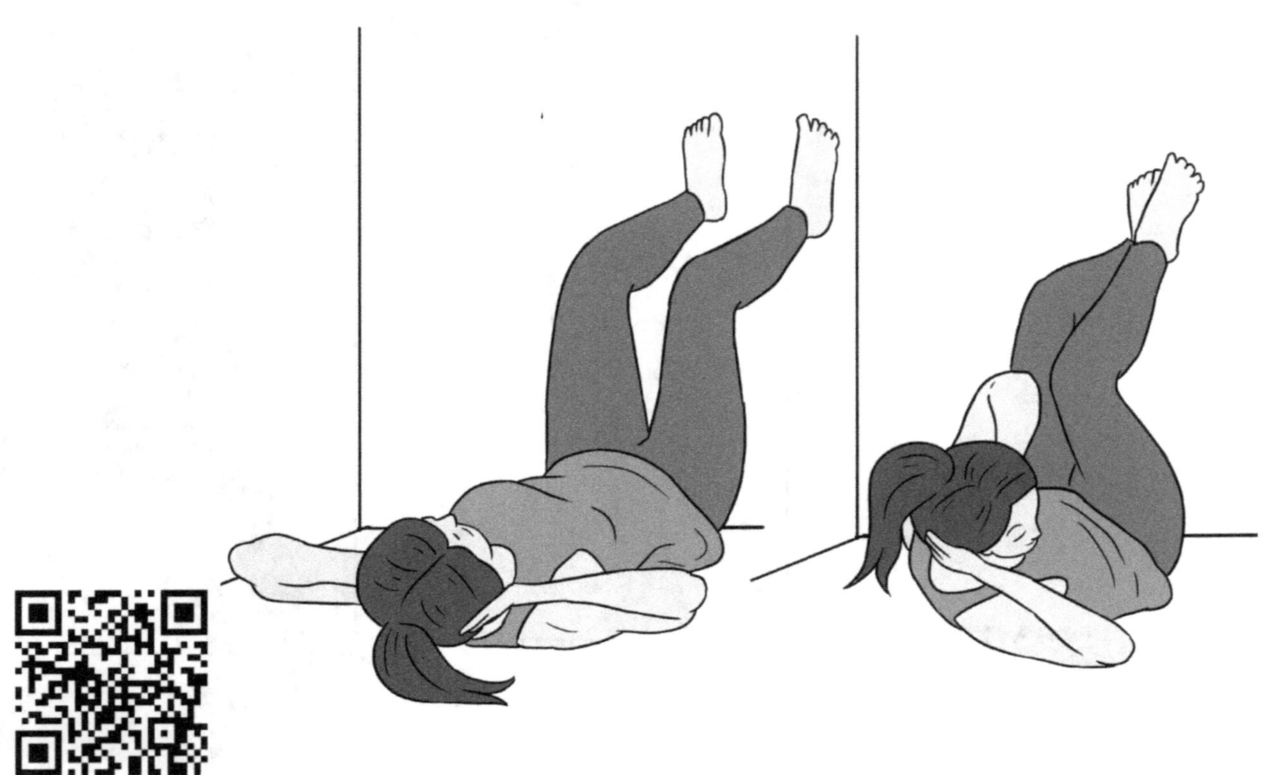

Instructions:

a. Lie on the back with hands behind the head and legs lifted, feet flat against the wall.

b. Rotate the torso and bring one elbow towards the opposite knee.

c. Switch sides in a fluid motion, as if pedaling a bicycle.

Safety Tips: Ensure the rotation comes from the core and not just the elbow. Keep the lower back pressed to the floor.

Repetitions: 10-12 reps on each side, 3 sets.

Wall-assisted Butterfly Stretches

Objective: To improve flexibility in the inner thighs and hips.

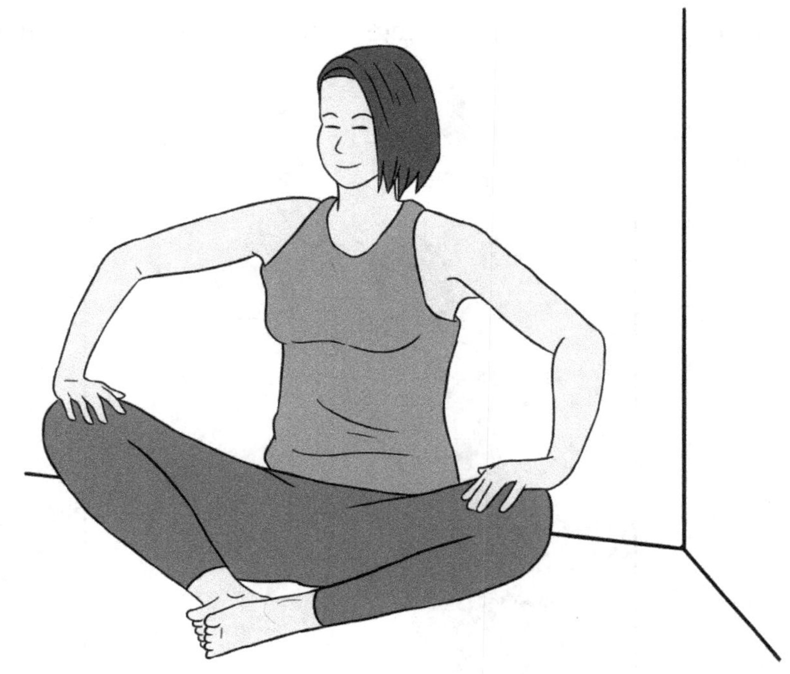

Instructions:

a. Sit on the floor with your spine straight, bringing the soles of your feet together.

b. Move your heels close to your pelvis.

c. Lean back slightly and place your hands on the wall behind you for support.

d. Gently press your knees down towards the floor, feeling a stretch in the inner thighs.

e. Hold the stretch for a few moments, then release.

Safety Tips: Ensure your back remains straight. If you feel any pain, ease out of the stretch.

Repetitions: Hold for 20-30 seconds, 3 times.

Wall Sliders
(using cloth or paper plates)

Objective: To challenge the core, legs, and glutes in a controlled sliding motion.

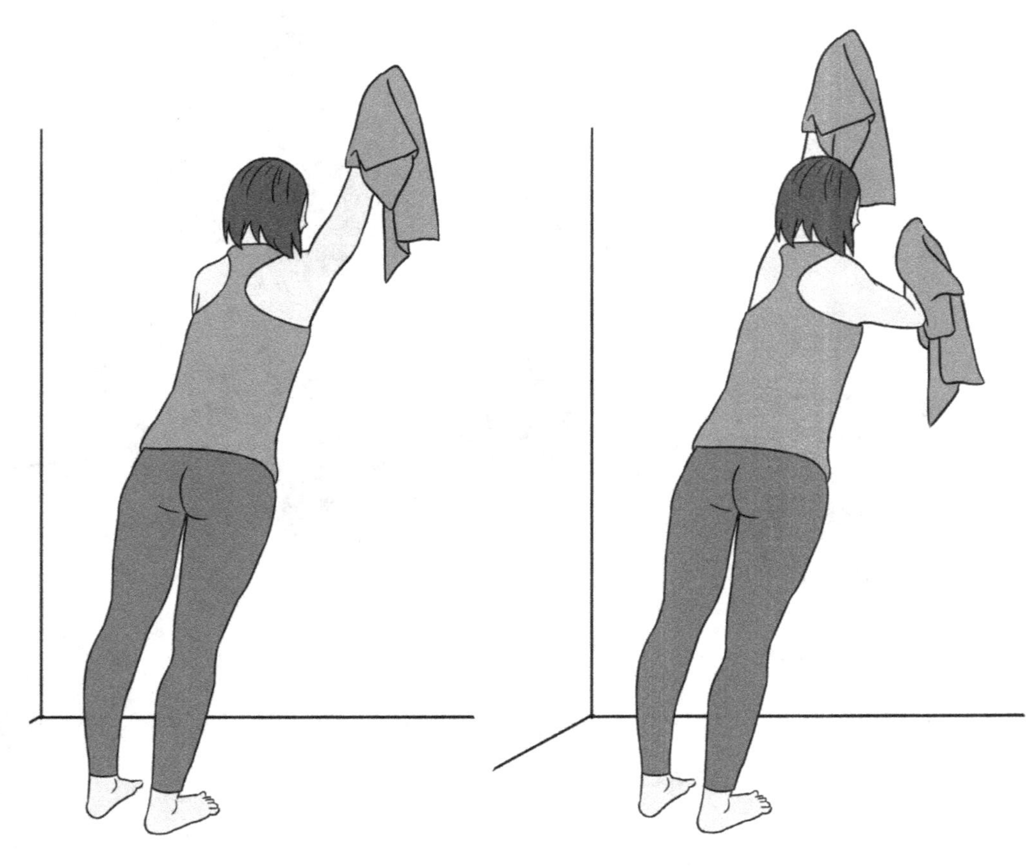

Instructions:

a. Start in a plank position facing away from the wall, hands on the floor, and feet on cloths or paper plates.

b. Engage the core and slide your feet up the wall, bringing the knees towards the chest.

c. Slowly slide back down to the starting plank position.

d. Repeat the movement for the set duration.

Safety Tips: Keep the core tight and avoid arching the back.

Repetitions: 10-12 reps, 2-3 sets.

Wall-assisted Pilates Saw

Objective: To stretch and strengthen the spine, shoulders, and obliques.

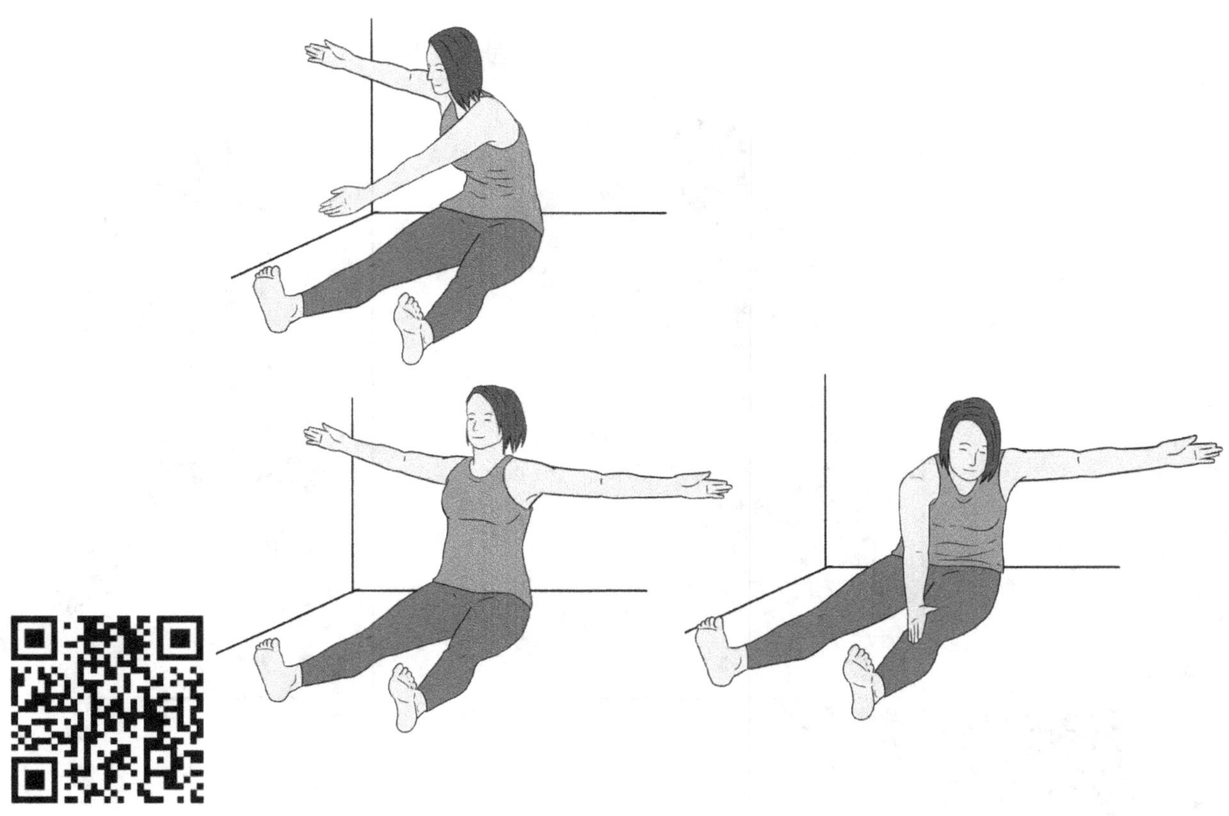

Instructions:

a. Sit on the floor with legs spread wide and feet against the wall.

b. Extend arms out to the sides at shoulder height.

c. Rotate the upper body to the right, reaching the left hand towards the right foot.

d. Look towards the back hand while doing so.

e. Return to the center and switch sides.

Safety Tips: Ensure the movements are controlled and avoid any jerky motions.

Repetitions: 8 reps on each side, 2-3 sets.

Wall Plank with Leg Abduction

Objective: To strengthen the core and work on the outer thighs and glutes.

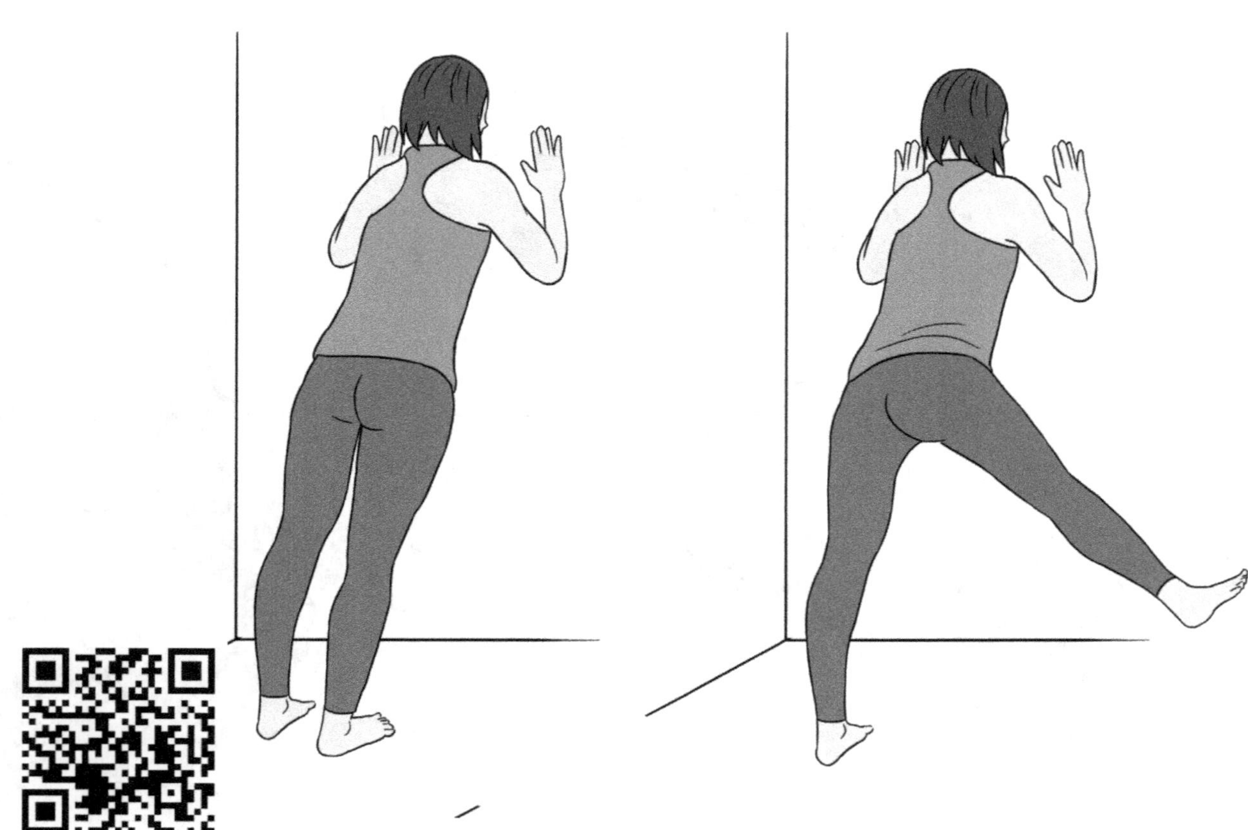

Instructions:

a. Begin in a plank position facing away from the wall, with feet resting against its base.

b. Engage the core and lift the right leg away from the wall in a sideward motion.

c. Return the right leg to the starting position.

d. Repeat the movement with the left leg.

Safety Tips: Maintain a solid plank position throughout. Keep the lifted leg straight.

Repetitions: 10 reps on each side, 2-3 sets.

Wall-assisted Russian Twists

Objective: To target the obliques, strengthen the core, and improve rotational mobility.

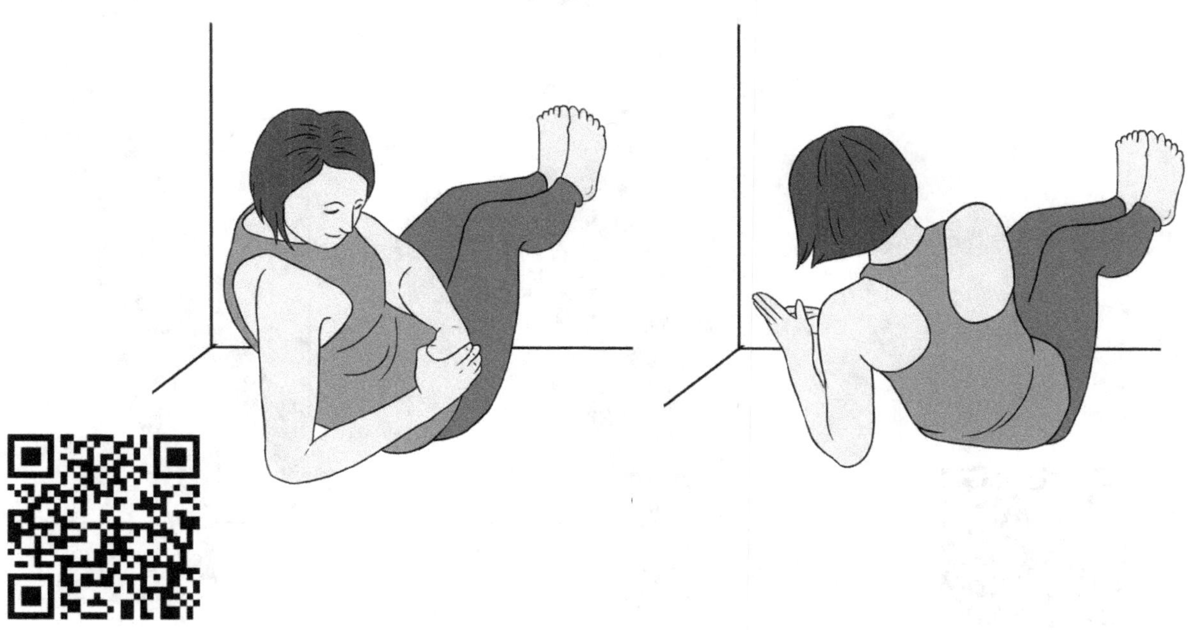

Instructions:

a. Sit on the floor with the soles of your feet pressed against the wall, knees bent.

b. Lean back slightly, creating a V-shape with the upper body and thighs.

c. Clasp hands together in front of the chest.

d. With a straight back, rotate the torso to the right, aiming to bring the hands beside the hip.

e. Return to the center and then rotate to the left. f. Continue alternating sides.

Safety Tips: Keep the spine long and straight. Ensure the movement is controlled and avoid using momentum.

Repetitions: 12-15 reps on each side, 2-3 sets.

Advanced Wall Side Plank with Leg Lift

Objective: To challenge the obliques, hips, and shoulders, fostering balance and core strength.

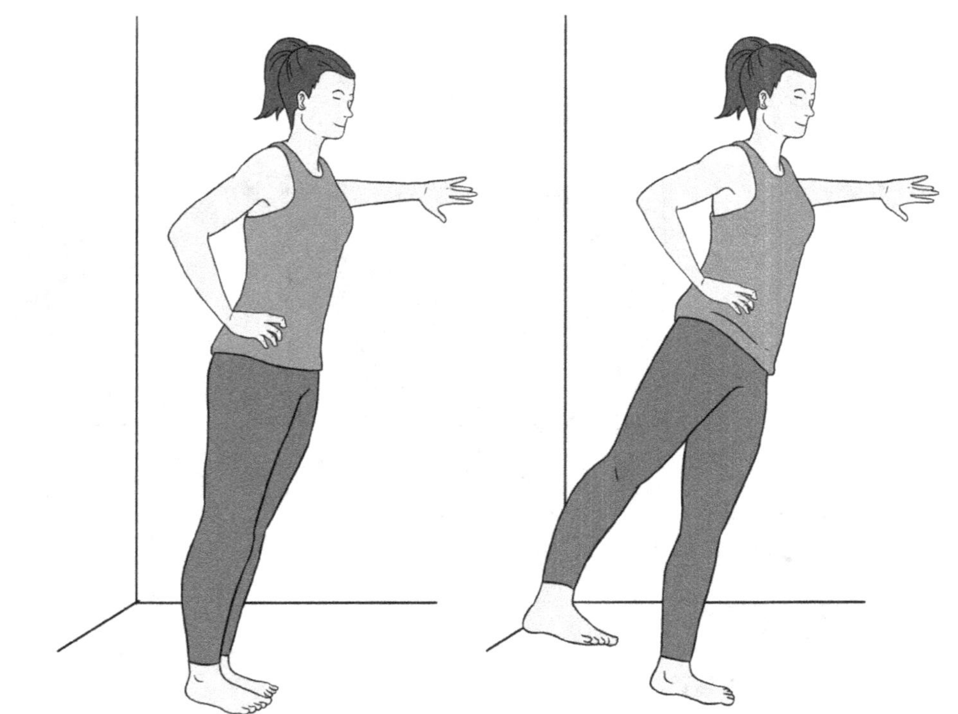

Instructions:

a. Begin in a side plank position with the left forearm on the floor and the soles of the feet pressed against the wall.

b. Keep the body in a straight line from head to heels.

c. Lift the top leg (right leg) upwards as high as comfortably possible.

d. Lower the leg back to starting position.

e. Repeat for the set number of repetitions and then switch sides.

Safety Tips: Ensure the supporting shoulder is stacked above the elbow. Engage the core throughout.

Repetitions: 10 reps on each side, 2-3 sets.

Every exercise is more than just a movement; it's a message to the body. It tells the body that despite challenges, it can adapt, grow, and conquer. The wall, a simple yet effective tool, assists in these advanced exercises, transforming them into powerful routines. It offers support when needed, resistance when desired, and a guide for alignment.

These advanced exercises, while demanding, are also rewarding. They're a testament to the power of Pilates and its ability to shape not just the body but also the mind. With every rotation, pulse, and dive, there's a deeper connection formed – a connection between movement and breath, body and mind, challenge and accomplishment.

The beauty of Wall Pilates lies in its simplicity. A wall, some dedication, and the right exercises can lead to transformations that are both visible and felt. These exercises, while advanced, are achievable. They require patience, persistence, and a dash of bravery. But with each repetition, they remind us that limits are often just in our minds and that with the right support and guidance, anything is possible. So, go on and challenge yourself, knowing that with every move, you're one step closer to a stronger, more flexible, and balanced self.

Chapter 11
Your Personalized Wall Pilates Prescription

Wall Pilates is such a gem. While its foundational principles remain consistent, the beauty of this practice is its adaptability. Everyone comes with a unique set of physical challenges, be it a sore back, creaky joints, or the weight of stress bearing down on their shoulders. Recognizing this, wall Pilates offers a range of exercises, each designed to address specific concerns.

This chapter is dedicated to personalizing your wall Pilates experience. It's like having a bespoke suit, crafted to fit you perfectly. Whether you're battling back pain after long hours at the office, dealing with joints that voice their displeasure a bit too loudly, or seeking a refuge from the whirlwind of daily stresses, there's a wall Pilates prescription waiting for you.

Let's dive in and explore these tailored routines, ensuring that your wall Pilates practice becomes as unique as you are, catering precisely to your needs. This isn't just about fitness; it's about crafting a personal wellness narrative that echoes with your individual challenges and triumphs. Welcome to the world of personalized wall Pilates.

Sore Back? We've Got Your Back!

Back pain is akin to an uninvited guest that overstays its welcome. Many face the discomfort of a sore back, whether it arises from long hours at a desk, lifting heavy objects, or simply the wear and tear of daily life. A sore back can be a constant nagging companion, making even the simplest of tasks seem daunting. But there's hope on the horizon, and it comes in the form of wall Pilates.

The Anatomy of Back Pain

The human back is a complex structure made up of bones, muscles, and connective tissues. It carries the weight of the body, provides support, and enables a wide range of movements. Given its crucial role, it's no surprise that the back is prone to discomfort and pain.

Back pain can have various origins. It might be muscular, stemming from strain or overuse. Sometimes, it's the spine's discs, which act as cushions between the vertebrae, causing the pain. Aging, poor posture, and even stress can also contribute to back discomfort.

Wall Pilates: The Natural Solution

Wall Pilates offers exercises that focus on strengthening the core. Now, one might wonder, what does the core have to do with the back? A lot, actually. A strong core provides better support to the spine, reducing the strain on the back muscles. When the core muscles are weak, the back muscles have to pick up the slack, leading to overuse and, eventually, pain.

The exercises in wall Pilates also emphasize alignment and posture. Proper posture ensures that the weight of the body is distributed evenly, preventing undue pressure on any particular part of the back.

Exercises Tailored for Back Relief

Wall Pilates offers a range of exercises that can be particularly beneficial for those with a sore back. Here are a few:

Wall Roll Down: This exercise stretches the entire spine, providing relief from stiffness. It also activates the core, promoting strength.

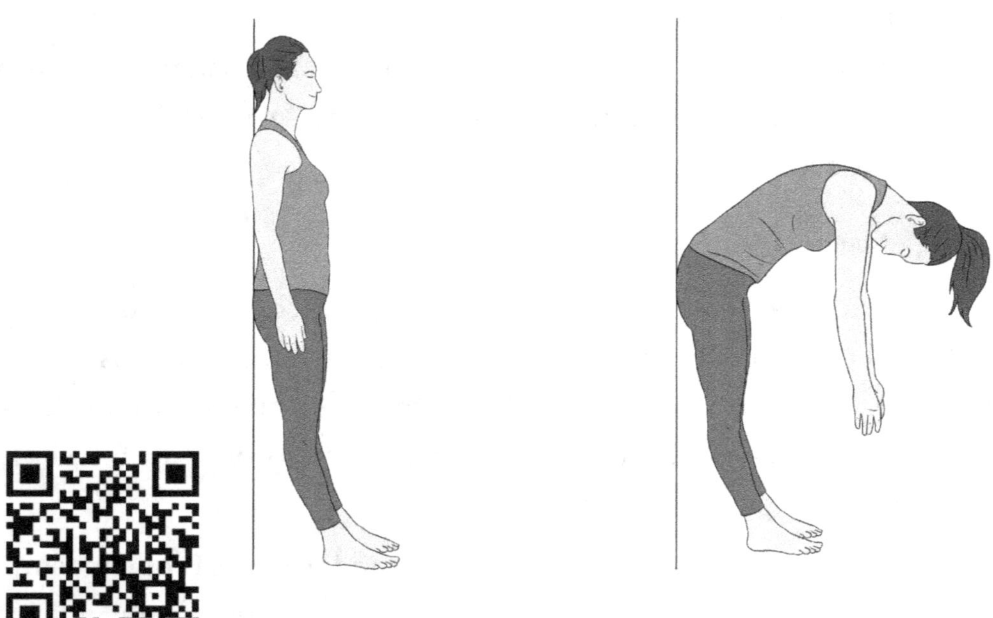

- **Start:** Stand with your back to the wall, feet hip-width apart, a few inches from the wall. Keep your spine straight, shoulders down, arms by your sides.
- **Initiate Roll Down:** Nod your head forward, starting the roll down with your chin toward your chest.
- **Roll Down:** Curve your back forward from top to bottom, letting your arms hang. Peel your spine away from the wall, vertebra by vertebra, knees slightly bent.
- **Forward Bend:** Continue until your hands are near the floor, maintaining a slight knee bend. Relax your neck.
- **Roll Up:** Reverse the motion, starting with your tailbone and rolling up slowly, straightening each part of your back, finishing with your head.
- **Adjust:** Stand tall, roll your shoulders back to relax them, and breathe deeply to reset your posture.

Wall Plank: A plank against the wall engages the core muscles, strengthening them and providing better support to the back.

Leg Slides: This exercise, done with the back against the wall, ensures that the spine remains neutral, preventing any arching that might cause strain. It also activates the deep abdominal muscles, which are essential for spine support.

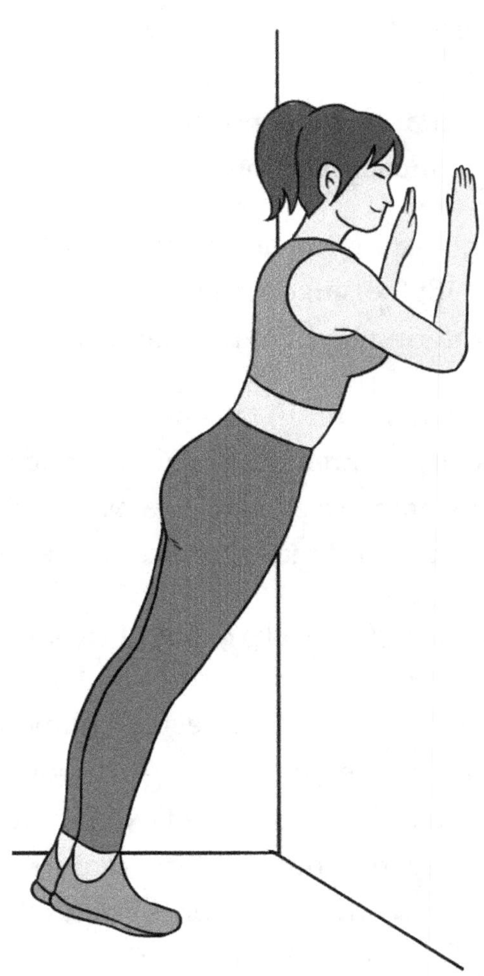

The Benefits Extend Beyond Pain Relief

While the primary goal might be pain relief, wall Pilates offers so much more. Improved flexibility, better posture, and increased awareness of body alignment are just some of the added benefits. Over time, with regular practice, one might find that not only is the pain reduced, but there's also an overall improvement in physical well-being.

Additionally, wall Pilates provides a space for relaxation. The focus on controlled breathing and movement can be meditative, offering a break from the stresses of daily life. This relaxation can, in turn, contribute to back pain relief, as stress is often a contributing factor to muscle tension and pain.

A sore back can be limiting, casting a shadow over daily activities. But it doesn't have to be a life sentence. With tools like wall Pilates, there's a way out. It's a gentle yet effective approach, offering both immediate relief and long-term benefits.

So, for those plagued by back discomfort, take heart. Wall Pilates is here, ready to offer its support. With its focus on strength, alignment, and overall well-being, it's the perfect companion on the path to a pain-free back. It's a promise of better days, where the back is strong, supple, and ready to take on the world.

Joints Acting Up? Try These

Our bodies are marvels of engineering, with every component playing a crucial role in ensuring smooth operations. Joints, the pivot points where bones meet, are vital players in this system, granting us the flexibility to move freely. Yet, for many, these very joints can become sources of discomfort and pain. Whether it's the creaky knees that protest every morning or the stiff elbows that resist movement, joint issues can be a hindrance. However, with the magic of wall Pilates, there's a way to soothe these aches and ensure that the joints remain supple and functional.

The Story Behind Joint Pain

Joints are complex structures, composed of bone ends cushioned by cartilage, all enclosed in a capsule filled with synovial fluid. This fluid acts as a lubricant, ensuring smooth movement. Over time, due to factors like aging, wear and tear, or injuries, the cartilage can wear down. This leads to bones rubbing against each other, causing discomfort.

Another common cause of joint pain is inflammation, often seen in conditions like arthritis. The inflamed joint can be swollen, warm to the touch, and painful, limiting movement.

Wall Pilates: The Gentle Approach to Joint Health

Wall Pilates comes into the picture as a gentle yet effective method to address joint issues. Here's how:

- **Low Impact**: The exercises in wall Pilates are low impact, meaning they don't put undue stress on the joints. This is especially beneficial for those already experiencing joint discomfort.
- **Range of Motion**: Wall Pilates exercises often involve moving the joints through their full range of motion. This helps in maintaining and even improving joint flexibility.
- **Strengthening Surrounding Muscles**: Strong muscles provide better support to joints. Wall Pilates targets various muscle groups, ensuring that joints are well-supported and protected from strain.

Specific Exercises for Joint Relief

Wall Pilates offers a plethora of exercises that can be particularly beneficial for those with joint issues. Here are a few to consider:

Wall Angels: This exercise is excellent for shoulder joints. By moving the arms up and down against the wall, it promotes flexibility and strength in the shoulder region.

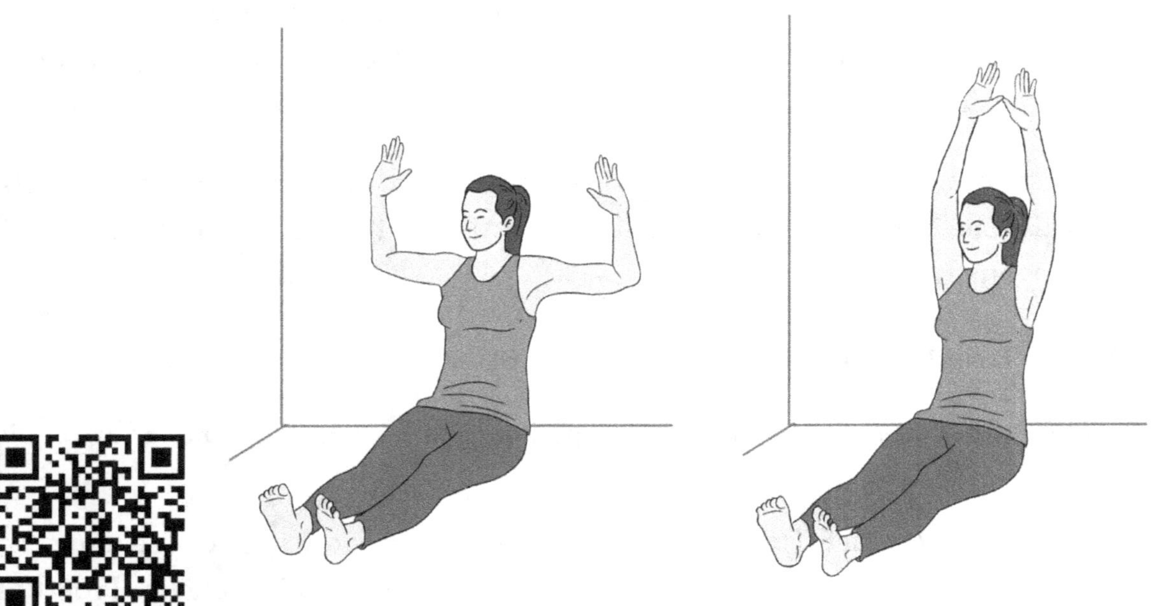

Start Position: Sit with your back against a wall, legs extended in front of you or knees bent with feet flat on the floor, depending on your flexibility and comfort. Ensure your lower back, upper back, shoulders, and head are pressed against the wall.

Arm Position: Lift your arms to the sides with elbows bent, forming a "W" shape with your body. Your arms, including the backs of your hands and elbows, should touch the wall.

Movement: Slowly slide your arms upward, maintaining contact between your arms and the wall, as if creating snow angels. Extend as far as possible while keeping your back and arms against the wall.

Return: Lower your arms back to the initial "W" position, keeping them in contact with the wall throughout the movement.

Repetitions: Perform 2-3 sets of 8-10 repetitions each.

Wall Sits: Beneficial for the knee joints, this exercise strengthens the thigh muscles, providing better support to the knees.

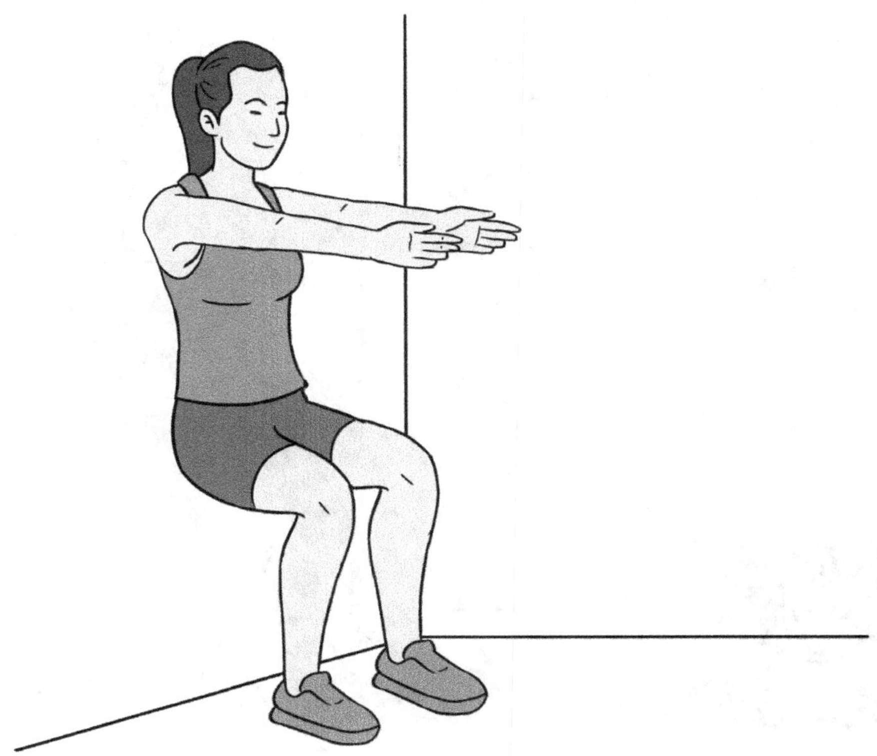

Leg Circles: This exercise targets the hip joints, promoting flexibility and strength in the surrounding muscles.

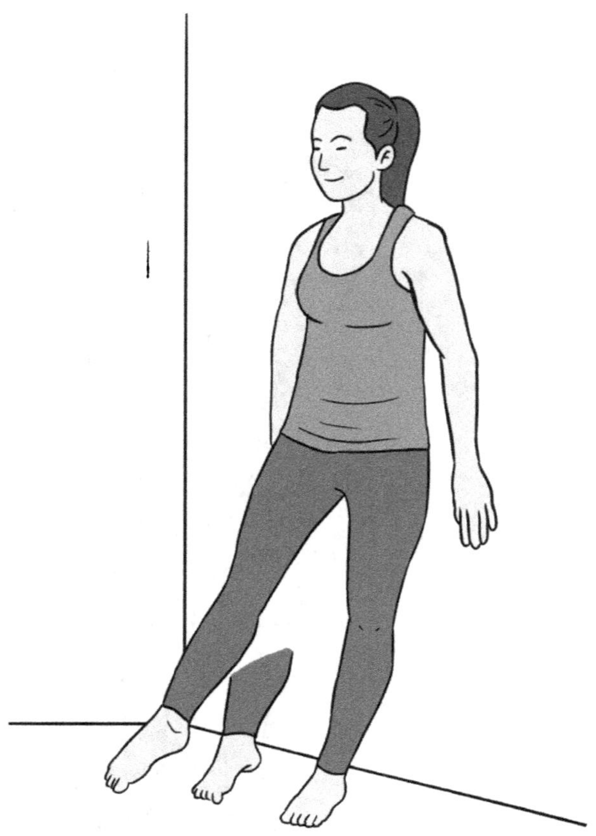

Start: Stand with your back and head against the wall, feet hip-width apart, ensuring a straight spine.

Leg Prep: Tighten your core, press your lower back to the wall, and lift one leg straight out. Bend the knee slightly if needed.

Circle Movement: Make small leg circles, gradually increasing size for control. Focus on smooth hip-driven movements.

Reps and Direction: Do 5-10 circles in each direction, keeping your movements controlled and back flat against the wall.

Switch: Lower the leg and repeat with the other leg, maintaining form and stability.

Beyond Just Exercise

While the primary focus of wall Pilates is on physical exercises, it's essential to acknowledge its holistic approach. The emphasis on controlled breathing, for instance, can help in managing pain. Deep, mindful breathing can act as a natural painkiller, relaxing the body and reducing muscle tension.

Additionally, wall Pilates promotes body awareness. With regular practice, one becomes more attuned to their body's signals. This awareness can help in identifying potential issues early on, ensuring timely intervention and prevention of further complications.

Joints, with their pivotal role in movement, deserve care and attention. And while joint issues can be a challenge, they don't have to dictate the quality of life. Wall Pilates offers a path, a way to address these issues head-on without resorting to aggressive measures.

With its gentle exercises, focus on flexibility and strength, and holistic approach, wall Pilates promises a future where joints are not sources of pain but instruments of free, unhindered movement. It's a call to embrace movement, to celebrate the body's incredible capability, and to ensure that every joint, every pivot point, functions at its optimal best. So, for those joints that act up, there's now a solution, one that promises relief, strength, and a future filled with smooth moves.

Stressed Out? Wall Pilates to the Rescue

Stress is an inevitable part of life. From looming work deadlines to personal challenges, sources of stress are manifold. While short bursts of stress can act as motivators, pushing individuals to perform at their best, chronic stress can take a toll, both mentally and physically. Over time, unmanaged stress can lead to a host of issues including sleep disturbances, headaches, and even chronic illnesses. But amidst the cacophony of life's demands, there's a sanctuary waiting, offering respite and rejuvenation: Wall Pilates.

Understanding Stress

Stress is the body's natural response to challenges. When faced with a stressful situation, the body releases hormones like adrenaline and cortisol. These hormones prepare the body to face the challenge, a response often referred to as the 'fight or flight' mode. Heart rate increases, muscles tense up, and focus sharpens.

However, when stress becomes a constant companion, this once beneficial mechanism turns detrimental. The constant flood of stress hormones affects bodily functions, leading to symptoms like fatigue, irritability, and even depression.

Wall Pilates: The Calming Influence

Wall Pilates offers a unique blend of physical exercises and mindfulness, making it a potent antidote to stress. Here's how it helps:

- **Mind-Body Connection**: Wall Pilates emphasizes the connection between the mind and body. Each movement is performed with awareness, drawing attention away from stressors and focusing it on the present moment. This acts as a form of meditation, calming the mind.
- **Deep Breathing**: Breathing exercises are integral to Wall Pilates. Deep, controlled breaths stimulate the parasympathetic nervous system, which counters the 'fight or flight' response, promoting relaxation.
- **Physical Activity**: Exercise, in any form, releases endorphins, the body's natural feel-good hormones. Wall Pilates, with its gentle yet effective movements, ensures a release of these mood elevators, providing immediate stress relief.

Specific Exercises for Stress Relief

While all Wall Pilates exercises offer some level of stress relief due to their inherent focus on mindfulness and breathing, some are particularly effective:

- **Wall Roll Down**: This exercise stretches the entire spine and allows a moment of relaxation at the bottom of the movement. The act of rolling down and then back up, combined with deep breathing, can be incredibly calming.

- **Leg Slides with Breathing**: Lying with the back against the wall and sliding the legs, synchronized with deep breaths, can be meditative. The repetitive movement and focus on breath draw attention away from stressors.
- **Wall-Supported Bridge**: Lifting the hips while the feet and shoulders are supported against the wall stretches the front of the body and engages the back muscles. Holding this pose and focusing on breathing can act as a stress-busting pause.

Beyond Just Exercises

The beauty of Wall Pilates lies in its holistic approach. Beyond the physical exercises, it fosters an attitude of self-care. Setting aside time for a session is, in essence, a commitment to oneself, a promise to prioritize well-being amidst life's chaos.

Furthermore, the principles learned during Wall Pilates sessions, especially the focus on deep breathing and mindfulness, can be applied to everyday situations. When faced with a stressful scenario, taking a moment to breathe deeply and center oneself can make a world of difference.

Stress, while unavoidable, doesn't have to rule life. With tools like Wall Pilates, there's a way to manage and even alleviate the pressures of daily living. It's a call to slow down, to tune into the body, and to find calm amidst the storm. With its blend of physical movement and mindfulness, Wall Pilates promises not just stress relief but also a renewed zest for life.

Wall Pilates offers just that, a sanctuary where stresses melt away, replaced by a sense of calm and well-being. It's more than just a fitness routine; it's a pathway to a balanced, harmonious life. So, when stress threatens to overwhelm, remember, Wall Pilates is here, ready to rescue and rejuvenate.

Chapter 12
Your 28-Day
Wall Pilates Plan

Three weeks might sound like a small window, but in the world of fitness and well-being, it can spark significant change. A consistent effort, even if just for a few weeks, can lay down the foundation for a lifetime of health and vitality. This chapter introduces a 28-day plan, handpicked and designed to guide individuals from the very basics of Wall Pilates to some more advanced moves.

The magic of this 28-day plan lies in its progressive nature. It's not about jumping into the deep end right away, but rather dipping one's toes, getting accustomed, and then diving deeper. Starting with 'Baby Steps' in the first week, the plan gently eases into 'Getting Serious' in the second week. By the time the third week rolls around, 'Showtime!' arrives with advanced moves and combinations to challenge the body in new ways.

Each day's exercise is selected with care, ensuring that the body gets a balanced workout throughout the week. From strengthening the core to improving balance and flexibility, the plan touches on various aspects of physical fitness. And the best part? All one needs is a wall and a dash of dedication.

In the world of Pilates, the wall isn't just a support structure. It's a partner, a guide, and sometimes, a challenger. It assists when needed and provides resistance when desired. This 28-day plan showcases the versatility of the wall in Pilates exercises. It's a journey from understanding one's body and its movements to pushing its boundaries.

Week 1: Baby Steps

Every great achievement starts with the decision to try. The initial days of any fitness routine are crucial. They set the tone, build habits, and provide the foundational strength that propels one forward. Week 1, aptly named "Baby Steps", is all about easing into Wall Pilates. It's a gentle introduction, ensuring that while the body is challenged, it's not overwhelmed.

The focus for this week is on understanding basic movements, getting a feel of the wall as a supporting partner, and building initial strength. The exercises chosen are simple yet effective, serving as a perfect entry point into the world of Wall Pilates.

Week 1: Foundation and Flexibility

Day 1:

✓	
	Wall Squat (10 reps)
	Wall-assisted Pelvic Tilts (12 reps)
	Wall Roll Down (8 reps)
	Wall Angels (10 reps)
I did it! ☺ ☺ ☺ ☺ ☺	

Day 2:

✓	
	Wall push-up (10 reps)
	Wall-assisted Toe Taps (15 reps each side)
	Wall Sits (30 seconds)
	Wall-assisted Dead Bug (10 reps each side)
I did it! ☺ ☺ ☺ ☺ ☺	

Day 3:

✓	
	Wall Bridge Preps (10 reps)
	Wall-assisted Knee Raises (12 reps each side)
	Standing Wall Circles clockwise (8 reps)
	Standing Wall Circles counterclockwise (8 reps)
I did it! ☺ ☺ ☺ ☺ ☺	

Day 4:

✓	
	Standing Wall-assisted Cat-Cow Stretch (12 reps)
	Wall-assisted Chest Opener Stretch (30 seconds hold)
	Leg Circles (10 reps each leg)
	Wall Clamshells (15 reps each side)
I did it! ☺ ☺ ☺ ☺ ☺	

Day 5:

✓	
	Wall-assisted Supine Leg Slides (12 reps each leg)
	Wall Plank Leg Slides (10 reps each leg)
	Wall-assisted Glute Bridges (12 reps)
	Wall T-push-ups (alternating sides) (10 reps each side)
I did it! ☺ ☺ ☺ ☺ ☺	

Day 6:

✓	
	Wall-assisted Seated Spine Stretch (30 seconds hold)
	Wall Supported Bridge (10 reps)
	Wall-assisted Leg Swings (front-back) (10 reps each leg)
	Wall-assisted Leg Swings (side-side) (10 reps each leg)
I did it! ☺ ☺ ☺ ☺ ☺	

Day 7:

✓	
	Wall Roll Down (8 reps)
	Wall Sits (45 seconds)
	Push-Ups Without Breaking a Sweat (12 reps)
	Wall Angels (12 reps)
I did it! ☺ ☺ ☺ ☺ ☺	

By the end of Day 7, the body should feel more flexible, stronger, and accustomed to the exercises. Each day's routine builds on the previous, preparing for the more intensive weeks ahead. The beauty of Wall Pilates is its adaptability, allowing each individual to move at their own pace, listen to their body, and enjoy the process.

Week 2: Getting Serious

With the foundation set in the first week, Week 2 is all about building upon that and challenging the body a tad more. The exercises in this week aim to push boundaries, but in a way that's enjoyable and not overwhelming. As the days go by, the body will become more familiar with the routines, making the process smoother.

Week 2: Strengthening and Stability

Day 8:

✓	
	Wall plank (30 seconds hold)
	Single-Leg Wall Squats (8 reps each leg)
	Wall-assisted Plank to Pike (10 reps)
	Wall-assisted Reverse Lunges (10 reps each leg)
I did it! ☺ ☺ ☺ ☺ ☺	

Day 9:

✓	
	Lunge Your Way to Greatness (10 reps each leg)
	Wall-assisted Superman Raises (12 reps)
	Standing Wall-assisted Torsion Control (8 reps each side)
	Wall-assisted Single Leg Deadlift (10 reps each leg)
I did it! ☺ ☺ ☺ ☺ ☺	

Day 10:

✓	
	Wall-assisted Arabesque (10 reps each leg)
	Wall Plank with Alternate Leg Lifts (10 reps each leg)
	Wall-assisted Starfish Sequence (8 reps)
	Wall-assisted Jackknife (10 reps)
I did it! ☺ ☺ ☺ ☺ ☺	

Day 11:

✓	
	Wall Side Plank (both sides) (30 seconds hold each side)
	Wall-assisted Scissors (12 reps each leg)
	Wall Plank Knee to Elbow (alternating sides) (10 reps each side)
	Wall Side Plank with Leg Lift (8 reps each side)
I did it! ☺ ☺ ☺ ☺ ☺	

Day 12:

✓	
	Spinal Rotation Stretch (30 seconds hold each side)
	Wall Roll Down (10 reps)
	Wall Plank Leg Slides (12 reps each leg)
	Wall Sliders (using cloth or paper plates) (10 reps)
I did it! ☺ ☺ ☺ ☺ ☺	

Day 13:

✓	
	Mountain Climbers (15 reps each leg)
	Isometric Wall Sit (60 seconds)
	Wall-assisted Pilates Saw (10 reps each side)
	Wall Plank with Leg Abduction (10 reps each leg)
I did it! ☺ ☺ ☺ ☺ ☺	

Day 14:

✓	
	Single-Leg Wall Squats (10 reps each leg)
	Wall-assisted Plank to Pike (12 reps)
	Wall Plank (45 seconds hold)
	Wall-assisted Reverse Lunges (12 reps each leg)
I did it! ☺ ☺ ☺ ☺ ☺	

As Week 2 nears its end, the intensity and complexity of the exercises have undeniably increased. However, with each passing day, the body's adaptability and resilience are also becoming evident. The routines are designed to challenge, but also to showcase the body's potential. With consistency, the results will not only be felt but also seen, making the effort all the more worthwhile.

Week 3: Showtime! Advanced Moves and Combos

As we dive into the third week, the exercises take on a more advanced tone. It's the week where all the foundational work from the preceding days comes to life in more complex and challenging forms. While these exercises may seem a bit daunting at first glance, it's essential to remember that the body has been adequately prepped and conditioned in the previous weeks. With focus, commitment, and a bit of grit, these exercises can be mastered.

Week 3: Advanced Techniques and Core Focus

Day 15:

✓	
	Wall Handstands (Partial) (5 reps)
	Advanced Wall Squat with Alternate Leg Lifts (8 reps each leg)
	Butterfly Stretches (30 seconds hold)
	Russian Twists (15 reps each side)
I did it! ☺ ☺ ☺ ☺ ☺	

Day 16:

✓	
	Wall Walks ((5 reps)
	Wall Roll-Ups (10 reps)
	Wall Plank with Rotation (8 reps each side)
	Pilates Teaser with Leg Extension (8 reps)
I did it! ☺ ☺ ☺ ☺ ☺	

Day 17:

✓	
	Wall Plank with Pulse (10 reps each leg)
	Swan Dive (10 reps)
	Criss-Cross (Pilates Bicycle) (15 reps each side)
	Wall Plank Knee to Elbow (alternating sides) (12 reps each side)
I did it! ☺ ☺ ☺ ☺ ☺	

Day 18:

✓	
	Wall Handstands (Partial) (6 reps)
	Wall Squat with Alternate Leg Lifts (10 reps each leg)
	Butterfly Stretches (35 seconds hold)
	Russian Twists (18 reps each side)
I did it! ☺ ☺ ☺ ☺ ☺	

Day 19:

✓	
	Wall Walks (6 reps)
	Wall Roll-Ups (12 reps)
	Wall Plank with Rotation (10 reps each side)
	Pilates Teaser with Leg Extension (10 reps)
I did it! ☺ ☺ ☺ ☺ ☺	

Day 20:

✓	
	Single-Leg Wall Plank with Pulse (12 reps each leg)
	Wall-assisted Swan Dive (12 reps)
	Wall-assisted Criss-Cross (18 reps each side)
	Wall Plank Knee to Elbow (14 reps each side)
I did it! ☺ ☺ ☺ ☺ ☺	

Day 21:

✓	
	Mountain Climbers (18 reps each leg)
	Isometric Wall Sit (75 seconds)
	Wall-assisted Pilates Saw (12 reps each side)
	Wall Plank with Leg Abduction (12 reps each leg)
I did it! ☺ ☺ ☺ ☺ ☺	

Week 4: Integration and Mastery

It's time to bring everything together, pushing for mastery over the complex exercises you've learned. This week challenges your strength, technique, and mental grit, emphasizing the harmony between your body and mind. Celebrate your progress, refine your movements, and let's finish strong. Ready to conquer the last stretch? Let's make it count!

Day 22:

✓	
	Arabesque (12 reps each leg)
	Wall Side Plank (both sides) (35 seconds hold each side)
	Superman Raises (15 reps)
	Standing Wall-assisted Torsion Control (10 reps each side)
I did it! ☺ ☺ ☺ ☺ ☺	

Day 23:

✓	
	Seated Spine Stretch (35 seconds hold)
	Wall Supported Bridge (12 reps)
	Swings (front-back) (12 reps each leg)
	Leg Swings (side-side) (12 reps each leg)
I did it! ☺ ☺ ☺ ☺ ☺	

Day 24:

✓	
	Wall Roll Down (12 reps)
	Wall Sits (50 seconds)
	Push-Ups Without Breaking a Sweat (15 reps)
	Wall Angels (15 reps)
I did it! ☺ ☺ ☺ ☺ ☺	

Day 25:

✓	
	Wall Plankl! (50 seconds hold)
	Single-Leg Wall Squats (12 reps each leg)
	Plank to Pike (15 reps)
	Reverse Lunges (15 reps each leg)
I did it! ☺ ☺ ☺ ☺ ☺	

Day 26:

✓	
	Wall Handstands (Partial) (7 reps)
	Wall Squat with Alternate Leg Lifts (12 reps each leg)
	Butterfly Stretches (40 seconds hold)
	Russian Twists (20 reps each side)
I did it! ☺ ☺ ☺ ☺ ☺	

Day 27:

✓	
	Wall Walks (7 reps)
	Wall Roll-Ups (15 reps)
	Wall Plank with Rotation (12 reps each side)
	Rest
I did it! ☺ ☺ ☺ ☺ ☺	

Day 28:

✓	
	Single-Leg Wall Plank with Pulse (15 reps each leg)
	Swan Dive (15 reps)
	Criss-Cross (20 reps each side)
	Wall Plank Knee to Elbow (16 reps each side)
I did it! ☺ ☺ ☺ ☺ ☺	

Concluding the 28-day Wall Pilates plan, these final exercises serve as a testament to progress, a celebration of the strength garnered, and the flexibility achieved. Every twist, plank, and extension reflect not just physical capability but also mental resilience and dedication. Remember, the wall, throughout this journey, has been more than just a prop; it's been a silent partner, reflecting every push and every pull. As the days end, take a moment to appreciate the transformation, both seen and unseen. And as the heart beats and the breath flows, know that this is just the beginning of many more challenges to conquer and peaks to scale.

Chapter 13
Frequently Asked Questions

Whenever we embrace something new, a flurry of questions often fills our minds. It's a natural part of the learning curve and aids in understanding and adapting. Wall Pilates, while simple and effective, can be a novelty for many. Whether it's the curious beginner or the seasoned fitness enthusiast considering a fresh approach, everyone has questions. This chapter aims to shed light on some of the most common queries about Wall Pilates. From its universal suitability to what to do if a session is missed, let's unravel the answers and make the Wall Pilates experience even more rewarding.

Is Wall Pilates a Good Fit for Everyone?

When we think of fitness, we often picture a gym packed with equipment or perhaps an open field where people jog, leap, and stretch. But not all exercises require such space or gear. Enter Wall Pilates, a unique method that leverages the sturdiest "equipment" in your home: the wall. As its popularity rises, a pressing question emerges: Is it suitable for everyone?

A Universal Design

Wall Pilates offers an exciting twist on traditional Pilates by integrating the support and resistance of a wall. This design inherently makes the exercises more accessible. For those who might find floor exercises challenging, the wall provides a stable platform, reducing the strain on joints and muscles. This means that people of various age groups, from energetic teenagers to active seniors, can benefit from this form of exercise.

Beginners Welcome

For those new to the world of fitness or Pilates, the wall acts as a comforting companion. It offers support, allowing beginners to familiarize themselves with movements without feeling overwhelmed. The risk of incorrect postures is minimized, as the wall guides the body, ensuring alignment and balance. As confidence builds, one can gradually progress, increasing the intensity and complexity of exercises.

Adaptable for the Experienced

But what about those who already have a strong fitness foundation? For the seasoned exerciser, Wall Pilates is far from boring. By playing with angles, resistance, and incorporating props like resistance bands or light weights, the exercises can be amplified to challenge even the most experienced individuals. This adaptability ensures that Wall Pilates remains engaging, pushing individuals to new limits while still being safe.

Considerations for Special Populations

While Wall Pilates boasts broad appeal, there are specific groups who should approach with caution or after seeking professional advice. Pregnant women, though they can benefit from the strengthening aspects of Pilates, should always consult with their healthcare provider before starting any new exercise regimen. Similarly, individuals with specific medical conditions, injuries, or post-surgery should discuss with a physiotherapist or medical professional to ensure the exercises won't exacerbate any issues.

The Psychological Benefits

Beyond the physical realm, Wall Pilates also extends its benefits to the mind. The concentration required to execute movements with precision, the breathing techniques integrated into exercises, and the sheer act of dedicating time to oneself, all contribute to mental well-being. People dealing with stress, anxiety, or simply looking for a mindful activity can find solace in the rhythmic movements against the wall.

The beauty of Wall Pilates is its genuine inclusivity. Whether someone is looking for low-impact exercises, rehabilitation movements, strength training, or simply a change from their routine, Wall Pilates has something to offer. Its simplicity doesn't diminish its potency. By allowing modifications, it caters to a spectrum of needs and fitness levels.

Is Wall Pilates a good fit for everyone? While the answer leans heavily towards a "yes," individual discretion based on personal health and fitness levels is always advised. However, its versatility, adaptability, and the minimal equipment requirement make it an attractive option for many. It breaks down barriers, making fitness accessible and enjoyable. So, if the question is about giving Wall Pilates a try, the wall is ready when you are. Just ensure to start slow, listen to your body, and enjoy the process.

Can You Overdose on Wall Pilates?

At first glance, the idea of "overdosing" on a form of exercise might seem a bit odd. How can something so beneficial become detrimental? As with most things in life, moderation is key. In the world of fitness, it's easy to assume that more is always better. Yet, the body, resilient as it is, also thrives on balance, rest, and variety. So, when it comes to Wall Pilates, a refreshing and innovative approach to traditional Pilates, how much is too much?

The Appeal of Wall Pilates

The magic of Wall Pilates lies in its simplicity. With no need for fancy equipment or large spaces, it's accessible and convenient. This convenience can be both a blessing and a curse. The wall, ever-present and always inviting, might tempt enthusiasts to engage in daily, lengthy sessions, thinking that more frequent and intense workouts will expedite results. But does this approach work, or could it be counterproductive?

The Body's Need for Recovery

Muscles grow and repair not during the workout, but during rest periods. Every time you engage in Wall Pilates, or any exercise for that matter, tiny tears form in the muscles. It's during rest that these tears heal, resulting in muscle growth. Overdoing Wall Pilates, especially without adequate rest, can interrupt this recovery process. This not only hampers muscle growth but also increases the risk of injuries.

Quality Over Quantity

It's easy to fall into the trap of thinking longer sessions equate to better outcomes. Yet, a focused 30-minute session, where each move is performed with precision and control, can be more beneficial than an hour-long session done hastily. Wall Pilates emphasizes alignment, core strength, and controlled movements. Rushing through exercises or doing them without proper technique reduces their effectiveness and can even lead to strain or injury.

The Mental Aspect

Physical repercussions aside, there's also a mental component to consider. Engaging in the same activity repetitively can lead to burnout. The initial enthusiasm might wane, replaced by a sense of obligation or even dread. By varying one's routine and incorporating other forms of exercise or activities, it keeps the mind engaged and the motivation levels high.

Signs You Might Be Overdoing It

While everyone's body is different, some universal signs indicate over-exertion:

Persistent Fatigue: Feeling tired even after a full night's rest.

- **Decreased Performance**: Struggling with exercises that were once easy.
- **Mood Swings**: Irritabili**ty or feelings of sadness.**
- **Sleep Disturbances**: Difficulty falling asleep or frequent waking during the night.
- **Chronic Soreness**: Muscles that ache for days after a workout.
- **Loss of Appetite**: Not feeling hungry or skipping meals.

If any of these signs are noticed, it might be time to evaluate and perhaps cut back on the frequency or intensity of Wall Pilates sessions.

Striking the Right Balance

For those starting with Wall Pilates, three to four times a week, with rest days in between, is a good rule of thumb. As one becomes more advanced, this frequency can be adjusted based on individual goals and how the body feels. Listening to one's body, taking rest days, staying hydrated, and ensuring a balanced diet are all crucial components of a holistic fitness approach.

While Wall Pilates is a fantastic addition to anyone's fitness routine, moderation is essential. It's not about how often or how long the sessions are, but how effectively and safely they're done. As with any good thing in life, balance is crucial. So, while the wall is always there, beckoning for another session, sometimes the best course of action might be to take a step back, rest, and then return with renewed vigor and enthusiasm. After all, fitness is a marathon, not a sprint.

Missed a Day? Here's How to Bounce Back

Life has an uncanny way of throwing curveballs. Whether it's an unexpected work commitment, an ill-timed cold, or simply the weight of daily tasks, there will inevitably be days when your Wall Pilates session gets pushed to the wayside. And that's okay. While consistency is important in any fitness regimen, it's equally essential to recognize that life isn't always predictable. The key isn't about never missing a day, but rather understanding how to get back on track when you do.

The Mental Hurdle

Often, the biggest challenge isn't the missed session itself but the guilt and self-reproach that accompany it. "I should have made time," "I'm letting myself down," "I'm never going to reach my goals at this rate" - these are common refrains that play in our minds. Yet, this self-talk isn't just unhelpful; it can be detrimental.

Firstly, understand that everyone has off days. Even the most disciplined athletes have moments when they need to rest or when other commitments take precedence. Rather than berating oneself, it's more productive to acknowledge the miss, understand the reason, and then move forward.

Don't Play Catch-Up

A common instinct after missing a Wall Pilates session is to make up for it by doubling the intensity or duration of the next workout. This approach might seem logical, but it can lead to burnout or injury. Your body expects a certain rhythm and pushing it suddenly can be counterproductive. Instead of trying to "make up" for the missed day, simply return to your routine as planned.

Reassess Your Schedule

If missing sessions becomes a pattern rather than an exception, it might be time to reassess. Perhaps your chosen workout time clashes with other commitments, or maybe the duration of each session feels too long given your current circumstances. There's no harm in tweaking your schedule or routine to better fit your lifestyle. Remember, the best workout is the one you stick with, so it's crucial to find a rhythm that feels sustainable.

Engage in Light Activity

On days when a full Wall Pilates session isn't feasible, consider light activities. A short walk, some gentle stretches, or even a few minutes of mindful breathing can keep you in the fitness mindset. These activities might not replace a Pilates session, but they help maintain a connection to your wellness goals.

Reframe Your Perspective

Instead of viewing a missed session as a setback, consider it a rest day. Rest is vital for muscle recovery, and sometimes, an unplanned break can be beneficial. It allows the body to recover fully, making your next session even more effective. Listen to your body; perhaps it needed that extra day of rest.

Remind yourself of why you started Wall Pilates in the first place. Whether it was to build strength, improve flexibility, or boost mental well-being, reconnecting with your goals can reignite your motivation. Consider keeping a journal to track your progress, jot down how you feel after each session, and note any improvements. On days when motivation wanes, looking back at your journey can provide the boost you need.

Seek Community Support

If you're finding it hard to bounce back after missing a few sessions, consider seeking support. Joining a Wall Pilates group, whether online or in person, can provide encouragement. Sharing your challenges and hearing others' experiences can offer both perspective and motivation.

Missing a Wall Pilates session, or even several, doesn't spell the end of your fitness journey. It's merely a slight detour. The path to wellness isn't a straight line; it's filled with ups and downs. What truly matters is your commitment to getting back on track, not the occasional missed step. After all, Wall Pilates, like life, is less about perfection and more about progress. So, the next time you miss a day, take a deep breath, let go of any guilt, and simply begin again. Your wall awaits.

Conclusion

Throughout the annals of history, walls have been symbols of many things-divisions, protection, art, and memories. Yet, in the realm of fitness, a wall is transformed, shedding its inert nature to become an active participant in our quest for health and well-being. Wall Pilates, as we have journeyed through its depths, has offered us a fresh lens to view not just the wall but our very relationship with fitness.

The principles of Wall Pilates are simple, yet their impact is profound. It's not about high-intensity workouts or complex routines but about understanding, connecting, and evolving. The wall, in its silent strength, offers support, resistance, and feedback. But more than that, it becomes a mirror, reflecting our progress, our challenges, and our triumphs.

As we explored the myriad benefits, from the sculpting advantages for women to the safety and support it provides seniors, and the vital role it plays in enhancing balance and stability, a pattern emerged. Wall Pilates isn't just about physical transformation. It's a holistic approach, touching every facet of our being - body, mind, and soul.

Our modern world, with its relentless pace and constant demands, often leaves little room for introspection, for truly connecting with oneself. Here, Wall Pilates stands as a sanctuary. Each session, each movement against the wall, becomes a moment of pause, a respite from the chaos outside. The rhythmic motions, the push and pull against the wall, the deep breaths-all converge to create a symphony of self-awareness and peace.

It's also worth noting the beauty of inclusivity that Wall Pilates brings to the table. Fitness, often seen through the lens of age, ability, or even gender, finds a level playing ground here. The exercises, adaptable and modifiable, ensure that everyone, from a young adult to a senior, can find their rhythm, challenge their limits, and celebrate their progress.

But what truly stands out is the empowerment Wall Pilates offers. In a world filled with external metrics of success and well-being, Wall Pilates turns the gaze inward. Success isn't measured by how much weight one can lift or how fast one can run, but by how in tune one is with their body, by the joy of movement, and by the harmony between mind and body.